Chakras for Beginners

How to Balance Your Chakras, Radiate Energy and Heal Yourself

Copyright © 2015 by Tai Morello

Table of contents

Introduction 1

Chapter 1: The Subtle Body 4
  The Channels 5
  The Endgame of Spiritual Practice 7

Chapter 2: The Seven Chakras 10
  1. The Muladhara Chakra/ Root Chakra 11
  2. The Svadishthana Chakra / Sacral Chakra 12
  3. The Manipura Chakra / Navel Chakra 14
  4. The Anahata Chakra / Heart Chakra 16
  5. The Vishuddha Chakra / Throat Chakra 17
  6. The Ajña Chakra / Third Eye Chakra 19
  7. The Sahasrara Chakra / Crown chakra 21

Chapter 3: Balancing the Chakras 22
  Closing the Chakras? 22
  Identifying and Working on Imbalances 23

Chapter 4: Working with the Chakras 41
  Kundalini 42
  Hatha Yoga 42
  Pranayama 43
  Visualization 47
  Sounding the Seed Syllables 51
  Essential Oils for the Chakras 52

Chapter 5: Healing the Chakras 53

Figuring Out the Problem 54

A Meditation to Heal the Wounded Chakras 56

Canal Locks 59

Healing the Chakras with Herbs 64

A Parting Word 70

Preview of Kundalini for Beginners 71

Preview of The Mindfulness Beginner's Bible 85

Introduction

If you've ever practiced yoga or learned about Eastern spirituality—or even if you're only familiar with a few pop-culture references—you've probably heard about chakras before. And *at least* you'll know that chakras are energy centers connected with certain parts of the body and the subtle energy moving through it.

This book is an introduction to a subject of exceeding complexity. It is neither an exhaustive account of the chakras, nor by any means the *only* account of the chakras. Although they might be known by other names, chakra-like systems—maps of the subtle body—are found in many cultures and spiritual traditions, from Indian Hinduism and Buddhist Vajrayana, to Chinese Taoism, Western esotericism, and even the Kabbalah.

But in this book, we'll be focusing on the Hindu system of seven chakras. It's not the only chakra system, and it's not even the only *Hindu* chakra system. Any number of chakras have been described—five, six, seven, twenty, even more. So to say the picture is complicated is an understatement.

There is even debate about whether the various chakra systems were meant to be descriptions of an *actual* subtle body with *actual* energy centers akin to physical organs, or if they were merely intended as guides to visualization for different kinds of meditation.

Still, in this book, we will treat the chakras *as if* they are actual components of a subtle body, even as we leave the overarching question of their existential status (physical? psychical? imaginal? fictitious?) unanswered. This agnostic approach means that you don't actually have to believe in the literal reality of chakras to get something out of this book and start working with the chakra system.

If you're interested in chakras in the first place, you're probably doing some kind of spiritual practice, such as yoga. But to get started with chakras, you don't have to buy into any particular religious point of view. You don't even have to believe that chakras exist. All you need are an openness to experimentation and the ability to use your imagination.

* * *

The general idea of any chakra system is this: your body contains a number of energy channels or *nadis,* some of them major and some minor. Different kinds of subtle energy (*vayu* or "wind") move through these channels, which affects both your body and mind. The points where the channels intersect in the body are called *chakras* (literally "wheels"). There are many chakras in the body, but the most well-known system outlines seven major ones.

This subtle energy system is subject to imbalances, which can cause physical, emotional, and spiritual disturbances both large and small. In particular, the chakras are vulnerable to blockages as well as overexcitation, so they need to be balanced. When all seven chakras are opened, the free flow of energy through them brings about spiritual awakening.

The idea of a subtle energy system in the body dates back to the Upanishads of the 7th or 8th century B.C., but the chakra system only really began to take its familiar form later, in the tantric period. There are many misconceptions about tantra in the West, chief among them the idea that it's all about sex. But tantra is less about better sex or a better orgasm than it is about working with one's embodied experience instead of trying to transcend the body, using the senses as a means to spiritual awakening rather than trying to block the senses. It involves a huge literature and an enormous body of meditative and yogic techniques, of which only a fraction involve sexuality.

Chief among the ideas in tantra is that the universe is the manifestation of the ultimate, divine reality. What that means in terms of the chakras is that your own body is a microcosm of the larger universe, and the divine energy that manifests the universe is also at work in the individual practitioner's body.

Working with the chakras can be tremendously liberating, but this approach is not without its dangers. Among other things, it can have unintended effects for your psychological well-being. That's why practices involving the subtle body are traditionally done with the close guidance of a qualified spiritual teacher who can correct any mistakes a student makes, see the blind spots of their ego, and help them steer safely clear of common pitfalls as well as resolve any problems that might come up. So if you find yourself wanting to get into the chakras more deeply as a result of reading this book, I strongly urge you to find a teacher who can guide you in your practice.

Chapter 1: The Subtle Body

If you've put in a significant amount of time on the meditation cushion, you've probably noticed that different emotions register in different places in the body. Falling in love, for example, can register as an expansive, light, warm sensation in the chest. And heartbreak is so called because of where we feel it, in our heart. Feeling suddenly moved to emotion might make us "choked up"—which we feel in our throat. A sudden disappointment or negative realization registers as a sinking feeling in our gut. In fact, what makes emotions distinct from thoughts is that we typically feel them as energetic events in the body. With a little introspection, we can easily see that our inner psychological life maps on to specific points in the body—the chakras.

The chakras are arranged vertically, from the base of the spine to the crown of the head. From bottom to top they are:

1. *Muladhara* or root chakra at the base of the spine
2. *Svadishthana* or sacral chakra, connected to the testes or ovaries
3. *Manipura* or navel chakra
4. *Anahata* or heart chakra, located not actually at the heart, but near it, in the center of the chest
5. *Vishuddha* or throat chakra
6. *Ajña*, the so-called "third eye," located behind the forehead
7. *Sahasrara* or crown chakra, located at the very top of the head

Each chakra is represented by a lotus flower with a certain number of petals, which are also characterized as the spokes of a wheel (*chakra*). These are actually minor channels branching off from the chakras. The chakras are connected to various physical functions and levels of human psychological and spiritual development—the mind, emotions, and higher levels of understanding. They are also connected to "seed syllables," or certain mantric sounds in Sanskrit, different colors, elements, and deities. Together they comprise a complete map of human existence, from our lowest functions to our highest potential.

The Channels

As I mentioned before, thousands of channels or *nadis* (72,000, to be exact), resembling veins or nerves, course through the subtle body. In terms of the seven major chakras, three channels are most important: the *shushumna*, the *ida*, and the *pingala*. The *shushumna* is the central channel, while *ida* and *pingala* are left and right, respectively, although they actually weave in and out of the chakras like a double-helical strand of DNA, so that sometimes the left channel *ida* is on the right, and the right channel *pingala* is on the left. The chakras are the seven places where all three channels intersect as *ida* and *pingala* criss-cross in their winding course.

- The *ida* is white in color. It's connected with the energy of the moon, the feminine principle, a cooling quality, and the Ganges River. In modern terms, it is also connected to the right hemisphere of the brain, commonly thought to be more intuitive, which governs the left half of the body. It terminates in the left nostril.
- The *pingala*, red in color, is connected with solar energy, the masculine principle, a heating effect, and the river Yamuna. It's connected with the brain's left hemisphere, which is rational and associated with linear thinking, and which governs the right half of the body. It terminates in the right nostril.

- The *shushumna* runs straight from the root chakra all the way to the crown, connecting all seven chakras. It has no color or attributes, but is completely transparent, like empty space. It is also the course that the *kundalini* energy, which lies latent or "coiled" like a serpent at the base of the spine, will take on its journey from the root chakra to the crown when it awakens, traversing each of the intervening chakras in turn. But for most of us, it remains dormant.

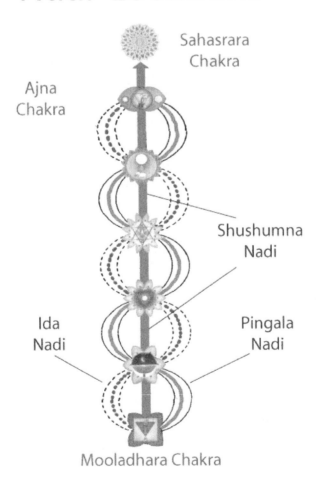

Ordinarily, we cycle back and forth between *ida* and *pingala*, usually with about an hour in each one. If you check against your own experience, you will notice that usually one of your nostrils is more open than the other one, and that is the main nostril through which you're breathing. For an hour, your breath will flow mainly through your left nostril, then the next hour through your right, and so on. But there can also be an imbalance between the two. That will register as an imbalance in the masculine and feminine modes of your psyche, or of the heating and cooling processes of the body. It could manifest as anything from sickness to emotional disturbance.

Balance is restored through a number of practices. But one of the main goals is to awaken the latent kundalini energy by stimulating it through exercises designed to move the energy of *prana* through *ida* and *pingala* in such a way that the kundalini rises through the central channel. If the energies enter into the central channel in the proper way, it can lead to rock-solid meditative stability and spiritual awakening. Your mind will become, like *shushumna*, transparent, spacious and crystalline.

So, in this system, methods like yoga and pranayama are employed to induce the energies to enter the central channel, where they will rise from the root chakra to the crown chakra, correcting any blockages or imbalances in the chakras along the way. That's the main goal of working with the chakras.

The Endgame of Spiritual Practice

Maybe it will be helpful at this point to say something about the ultimate spiritual goal of all this. From the point of view of this system, the ultimate reality of all things is one infinite, perfect, pristine consciousness. You could call this ultimate consciousness God, or the Self, or Being, or the Absolute. Maybe you'd be more comfortable with calling it the Tao, or even the Universe.

Let's not get hung up on semantics here. What we're talking about is an absolute point of changeless awareness or consciousness, a single still point which is the wellspring of all differentiated experience. It is nondual—it knows no distinction of subject and object, eternity and change, creator and creation. So it doesn't matter what you call it. The point is to realize that *Thou art That*—you are in some sense already identical with your primordial state, your true Self beyond the blind, limited "self" of ego.

All things find their unity in the absolute. This phenomenal world of plurality and variety that we experience with our senses is just an outpouring of divine energetic play. It is never separate from the ultimate unity of pure consciousness.

In tantra, this ultimate being is called Shiva. Shiva is the ultimate still point, perfect and changeless, the absolute awareness untouched by the vicissitudes of the world. The energy or power of Shiva issues forth as the endless dance of the phenomenal world. This energy is called Shakti, and she is thought of as Shiva's consort or wife. But in reality, Shiva and Shakti, the still point of pure awareness and the pulse and dynamism of life, are ultimately one.

Shiva is not some god "out there," but is only your own pure consciousness beyond time and space. Likewise, Shakti is not some external goddess, but is the energy and play of your own experience. As individuals, we are not separate from the absolute, but are merely its varied expressions, in just the same way that the waves on the surface of the ocean are one with that same ocean.

In terms of the subtle body, Shakti is the kundalini energy residing in the root chakra, while Shiva resides at the crown chakra. When Shakti awakens, she rises to meet Shiva at the crown chakra, and the two become one. That means that the dualistic back-and-forth of energy moving in the *ida* and *pingala* channels ceases, and their energies unify in the nondual *shushumna* channel.

Chapter 2: The Seven Chakras

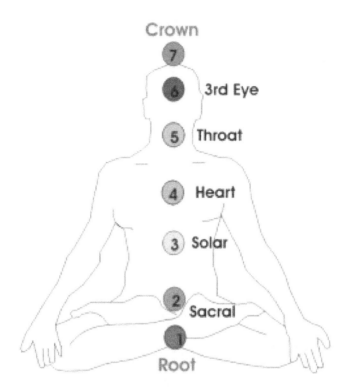

Now that we have an overall sense of what the chakras are, what their place is within the total ecology of the subtle body, and how that subtle body relates to the goals of spiritual practice, we're ready to look at the chakras and their qualities one by one.

1. The Muladhara Chakra/ Root Chakra

The first chakra is the *muladhara*, meaning "root basis," located at the base of the spine. The name itself supplies the clue to its significance. It is related to the basic physiological and psychological functions of the human organism—survival and instinct. As such, it has to do with security and survival-related activities, such as making money and procuring food. *Muladhara* is the foundation of the subtle body and the three main *nadis* of *ida*, *pingala,* and *shushumna*. It is also the location of the dormant kundalini.

The root chakra is visualized as a red, four-petaled lotus. As with the other chakras, each of the "petals" (sometimes "spokes") of the root chakra actually represents minor channels that branch out from it. So, in addition to the three major channels running vertically through the body, the root chakra also has four minor channels that branch from it, like veins or nerves.

Its element is earth. As this chakra is the root or foundation of the subtle body system, it is connected with the grounding energy of earth. An imbalance in this chakra might include feelings of insecurity, especially around financial matters, food, and shelter, which relate directly to physical survival. When the *muladhara* chakra is balanced, you feel safe, secure, and well-established in the solid quality of earth.

What this means is that, in order to work on the higher chakras and more developed areas of life, you need to first take care of your basic living situation. Have you got your life together in terms of money and a place to live? Psychologically, do you feel secure and safe, or do you suffer from worry about survival-related areas such as finances, job security, and so on?

This part of your life forms the root or basis for everything else, so if you don't take care of it first, the rest won't come together. If your root chakra is shaky, everything else—your sex life, social life, relationships, communication, intuition, and spirituality—will be shaky. It will all be thrown off because it's not resting on a secure foundation. So the lesson of the root chakra is: take care of your basic livelihood. Don't use spirituality or personal development as ways of avoiding your responsibilities.

The color of *muladhara* is red and its element is, unsurprisingly, earth. Earth, as an element in the system of five elements, is defined by its solidity. It is the support for everything that lives on it. Likewise, the *muladhara* chakra is the support of the chakra system, and our lives are built on its foundation. The seed syllable is *lam* (pronounced "lum"), which is the syllable of the earth element. Later in this book, when we talk about practices for activating the chakras, we'll explain the significance of the seed syllables.

2. The Svadishthana Chakra / Sacral Chakra

The *svadishthana* (SWAH deesh TAH nuh) chakra, or sacral chakra, is the second chakra, located at the coccyx or genital region, close to the root chakra and above it. The name *svadishthana* means "one's own abode." It is connected to the reproductive system and sexuality. Sexuality is very intimate, even private—hence the name, which suggests a highly personal situation.

Because it is related to sexuality, it is also related to the creativity and passionate energy of the libido. The desire related to *svadishthana* may be primarily unconscious. Since we're dealing with sexuality and the raw emotional energy of libido, we are talking about a somewhat wild, untamed kind of emotionality, hard to control. It can even manifest as cruelty. This is suggested by the *vrittis* associated with its six petals or subsidiary channels: affection, pitilessness, destructiveness, delusion, disdain, and paranoia. *Vrittis* are like disturbances in consciousness. Here, as with other chakras, they correspond to the minor channels that branch out from this chakra, and they manifest when energy moves through these channels.

The sacral chakra is represented by an orange-colored lotus of six petals. Its seed syllable if *vam*. Its element is water, a capricious element that takes many shapes, can be frozen or liquid, can flow swiftly and with great force or slowly and gently, or gather in one place and be still; it can erode surfaces or sustain life. The emotional quality of *svadishthana* is similarly multifarious, with tremendous creative and destructive potential.

Having worked on our basic living situation, we are ready to work on our emotional lives, starting with our passions and desires. The idea expressed by *svadishthana* is to balance the energy of our passions. Untrained and undirected, this energy can seethe beneath the surface of consciousness, erupting unexpectedly when somehow provoked. Working with *svadishthana*, we learn to harness this creative energy productively.

There are many reasons that the sacral chakra might be blocked or imbalanced. The trauma of sexual abuse is one reason. Another might have to do with repressed desires. The destructive potential of passion is threatening to society, which tries to control the way we express it. We each internalize this social superstructure in our own minds, and so learn to push troublesome feelings into unconsciousness.

So, while none of the chakras is particularly *easy* to work with, working with *svadishthana* might be especially volatile, as it can bring uppainful traumas and force us to confront oppressive conditioning. But it is necessary to make the effort if we hope to progress in our personal or spiritual growth. When this chakra is well-balanced, we know how to pursue and express our desires, including sexual desires, positively. We are not afraid of risks, but are able to ride our emotional energy to face new challenges. We are also in touch with our innate creativity.

3. The Manipura Chakra / Navel Chakra

Manipura means "city of jewels." This is the navel chakra, which is actually located slightly *above* the level of the navel. Its element is fire. Physically, it is connected to the metabolism and the "fire" of digestion, which transforms food, extracting its nutrients and processing the waste. Psychologically, it has to do with willpower, purpose, self-determination, fear, and anxiety.

The navel chakra is represented as a yellow, ten-petaled lotus. Its syllable is *ram*, the seed syllable of the fire element. Its function is transforming, burning, purposeful.

In Indian traditional medicine, digestion is likened to the burning of fire, which transforms fuel into heat and light and leaves ashes behind. Likewise, digestion transforms food, nourishing the body and contributing to its growth, giving it energy. It also leaves behind waste. The operation of one's personal agency in the world likewise has to do with transformation, shaping situations according to one's will.

If *svadishthana* has to do with the powerful energy of libido and passion, especially as expressed with an intimate other, *manipura* is more concerned with the exertion of one's willpower as a force of action in the public arena of society. Here the emotional energy is more developed and civilized than in *svadishthana*. It has found a mode of expression more suitable for the social world, as opposed to the raw, unprocessed emotionality of the sacral chakra, which finds its usual home in private situations.

In the root chakra we saw the basic survival instincts at work, in the sacral chakra the reproductive instinct. Here we see, for the first time, a more recognizably human quality, as opposed to what we have in common with animals. It is the emergence of a differentiated, human consciousness that sees itself as an independent agent pressing forward with its own agenda in the social sphere. So the key ideas around the *manipura* chakra include self-assertion, confidence, competition, exertion, will, and purpose.

When it is out of balance, it can manifest physically as poor digestion. Emotionally, an imbalance can come up in the form of excessive self-critical thoughts, timidity, fearfulness, lack of confidence—what some have called "paralysis of analysis." Or, on the other side of the imbalance, it can come up as a kind of pigheaded stubbornness, as with people who are overconfident and too forceful of their will. By activating and balancing the navel chakra, we can come to express our will in a confident and healthy way without stepping all over others.

4. The Anahata Chakra / Heart Chakra

The *anahata* or "unstruck" chakra is commonly called the "heart chakra," but this is a bit misleading. Although *anahata* is located close to the heart, it is actually in the center of the chest. There is a separate chakra, located slightly below and to the left of *anahata*, called *hrit*, literally "heart." But, as this is not considered a major chakra in the system we're presenting, we will carry on with the convention of calling *anahata* the "heart" chakra.

The name "unstruck" is curious, but it relates to the Vedic concept of the unstruck sound. That is the primordial, uncreated sound of *Om*, which is the universal vibration of all being. No one ever made or "struck" this sound, but it just sounds on its own, hence *anahata*. It is represented by a twelve-petaled lotus, green in color, with the seed syllable *yam*, which is the syllable of the air element.

As suggested by the name "unstruck," with *anahata* we are already moving beyond the realm of mundane thought and activity familiar to most of us, into the rarefied atmosphere of higher levels of being. *Anahata* is associated with feelings of love—not the intimate, erotic romance of lovers (that would be *svadishthana*), but universal, impartial love. You could call it compassion, or loving-kindness.

Unlike personal love, which often seeks to manipulate the beloved, the love we're talking about is not concerned with securing its own ground. It is quite selfless. It has no center because it has no ego, hence it is like the "unstruck sound" of *Om*—it just pervades everywhere equally and impartially.

We have seen the gradual development from the animal levels of survival and sexuality, to the human level of willpower, which is egoic. *Anahata* is starting to relate to a transpersonal, selfless level, which most of us never reach. So we can say that the heart chakra is the beginning of true spirituality.

An imbalance in the heart chakra can lead, physically, to respiratory disorders, heart disease, chest pain, and immune system disorders. Emotionally, it can manifest as a fear of being alone, bitterness, emotional unavailability, coldness, selfishness. Or we might be smothering in our love, trying to control our loved ones. These are the manifestations of neurosis at the level of the heart chakra.

When the heart chakra is balanced, we become generous, open, caring, and sensitive to the needs and feelings of others in a positive, not a neurotic way. The language we use is a dead giveaway: we say someone has a "big heart," or we talk about "opening one's heart." This is referring to the qualities of someone who has a well-balanced heart chakra.

5. The Vishuddha Chakra / Throat Chakra

The name of this chakra, *vishuddha* or *vishuddhi*, means "very pure." It's located in the region of the throat. It has to do with the power of speech, understood broadly here to mean the ability to communicate through any linguistic or symbolic means. That includes not just speaking and writing, but also the arts, which are symbolic forms of self-expression.

The first three chakras related to survival, sexuality, and willpower. The fourth chakra, at the heart, introduced a new mode of being not based on the manipulations of ego, but decentralized, impartial, and loving. Having developed that sense of love within ourselves, we discover that it longs to find expression. It needs a way of communicating itself.

The throat chakra is represented by a light-blue lotus with sixteen petals. The sixteen petals correspond to the sixteen vowels of classical Sanskrit phonology. The element connected with the throat chakra is space, and the seed-syllable of this chakra is the syllable of the space element, *ham*. The word for space in Sanskrit can also mean sky, so that is why this chakra is light blue in color.

Ordinarily, when we speak, we do so somewhat thoughtlessly. Sometimes we use speech in a manipulative way—to deceive others, or to sow discord. Or we use our words as weapons, to abuse and hurt. We may speak carelessly, not considering the impact our words might have on others. Thus vicious rumors can begin, simply because we wanted to entertain ourselves with conversation.

Vishuddha, the "very pure" chakra, enjoins us to maintain purity in the way we communicate. How we do so is suggested by the elemental nature of the chakra itself: we introduce space. Instead of letting words come out in a thoughtless rush, we speak them reflectively. We allow there to be a space between words and phrases, and we rest in that space for just a moment before we continue. In that way, we bring a meditative presence into our speech.

This manner of speaking mirrors the process of meditating on the breath. First there is an exhalation, which is like speech itself. The breath goes out and dissolves into space. Then, we breathe in. We don't hurry to suck breath back into our lungs so we can keep talking. The inhalation should be relaxed and comfortable, an opportunity to rest. Only then do we continue speaking.

An imbalance in this chakra can manifest as an inability to express yourself verbally. The inability to express yourself can be very distressing; it makes you feel powerless and voiceless. You have no way of making yourself heard. Alternately, you can misuse speech in the manner described above. Either way reflects that something is not right with the throatchakra.

When *vishuddha* is balanced, your speech comes naturally and easily. It has an easy-flowing, pleasant, and persuasive quality. You speak truthful, gentle, and timely words that are beneficial to others. If you are an artist, your art becomes an expression of your dignified mind and communicates a sane and kind perspective.

6. The Ajña Chakra / Third Eye Chakra

The sixth chakra, called *ajña*, is located superficially in the middle of the forehead, between and above the eyebrows. Internally, it is located at the pineal gland. It is often called the "third eye" because of its relation to seeing—not physical sight, but the insight of intuition. So we're talking about a special kind of knowing. The Sanskrit *ajña* means "command," as in the command of the teacher or guru. *Ajña* is the command center of the chakra system. It mediates between the higher self of the crown chakra and the rest of the chakras below it.

But it's also related to the word for knowledge, especially of a spiritual sort. We're still talking here about a differentiated kind of knowledge, not the highest knowledge of the absolute. This chakra is also connected to the faculties of imagination and dreaming.

Ajña is represented by a two-petaled lotus of a deep indigo color. *Ida* and *pingala* terminate here. Their duality reaches no higher than this level. It is associated with the mind element, and its seed syllable is *Om*, the primordial sound. Its presiding deity is Ardhanarishvara, a hermaphroditic form of Shiva-Shakti together. The union of male and female in one deity suggests that we are now approaching nonduality.

By the time we reach the level of the third eye, we have made contact with a sense of universal love and purified our speech. Now we have to develop a sense of wisdom. Without wisdom, our hearts might be expansive and loving, our speech might be pure in its intention, but we will still behave stupidly out of ignorance. We still have a chance to mess things up.

The insight of the third eye is not just some kind of psychic ability, although that is traditionally included here, as well. *Ajña* has to do with a penetrating vision that sees things completely and accurately. This insight is so sharp, so ruthless, that it penetrates through all illusion.

When the third eye chakra is imbalanced, it can lead to daydreaming, getting lost in a world of make believe, and even delusions and hallucinations. It's as if the calibration is off on our sensor. Or we may find ourselves rigidly attached to a belief system, religion, or ideology. Our thoughts and concepts become solid and inflexible.

When *ajña* is balanced and fully operational, the mind becomes extremely clear, perceptive, penetrating, and intuitive. It has a laser-beam focus that hits the point with exactitude. It easily sees through deception and manipulation, including the shifting self-deceptions of ego, and just as easily perceives the truth of things.

7. The Sahasrara Chakra / Crown chakra

The *sahasrara* chakra or "thousand-petaled" is called the crown chakra, and it's the pinnacle of the chakra system. It is said to be located either at the crown of the head, or in the space above it, depending on which tradition you consult.

As the name suggests, this chakra is represented by a lotus of one thousand petals. The petals are of many colors. The crown chakra is the ultimate white light, which refracts, as through a prism, into every color of the visible spectrum. There is no element connected with this chakra, nor a seed syllable. Instead, it is associated with the pure consciousness we mentioned before, the Absolute, which is identical to the highest Self. If it has any "element" at all, it is that of the ultimate voidness or emptiness, the ultimate unity beyond all attributes and qualities.

Sahasrara is both the source of all manifestation and the destination of spiritual striving. This chakra is the arrival point of the kundalini energy at the end of its journey. It is the residence of Shiva. When the kundalini reaches *sahasrara*, Shiva and Shakti, male and female, are united in the ultimate nondual state. At this point, one attains *nirvikalpa samadhi*, which is the complete identification of one's Self with the Absolute. This is enlightenment or awakening.

This chakra is inconceivable. It cannot be understood from an ordinary, dualistic point of view. Everything we say about it is mere metaphor, word, and image—a finger pointing to the moon, but not the moon itself. *Sahasrara* is the ultimate light of pure, nondual awareness.

Chapter 3: Balancing the Chakras

I'm sure you've probably heard about balancing the chakras and opening the chakras. Well, what do these phrases really mean? Given the hazards involved, it's good if we're about bit cynical about the idea.

One important thing to note is that balancing the chakras and opening the chakras are two different things. In the beginning, it's not a very good idea to try to blast your chakras wide open. Such an incautious approach will leave you vulnerable to unscrupulous people and negative energies.

Of course, the end goal of spiritual awakening is to open the chakras and to let kundalini energy flow throw them unimpeded. But that can only happen once you've strengthened your system. You need to beef it up a bit first, rewire the whole thing, because currently it can't take that level of voltage. Such a shock would just fry your circuitry, perhaps permanently.

Closing the Chakras?

So balancing the chakras is very important. It sounds a bit strange, but that might mean *closing* certain chakras that are too open—or at least closing them partially.

As I mentioned, there are bad people out there who will feed off your energy if you make yourself very vulnerable. They'll just suck you dry. Such people are called "energy vampires."

Additionally, there is a lot of pollution in our energetic environment. We get in the information we consume as much as the food we eat. And the air we breathe is a vector for polluted energy to enter our system. Since we absorb prana by breathing, pollution in the air can also contaminate our subtle body if it's too open to such influences.

Think of each chakra as like a house. If you leave the doors and windows wide open, thieves, murderers, and wild animals can come in and do as they please. On the other hand, if you bar the doors, shutter the windows, and lock yourself in like Boo Radley in *To Kill a Mockingbird*, then you shut yourself off from the world. Then you become a prisoner of your own paranoia—hardly a better way of doing things.

The balanced approach is to use your best judgment about which guests to invite into your home and which intruders to repel.

Identifying and Working on Imbalances

Before you try to balance your chakras, first you have to recognize where the imbalances are occurring. All that theory we covered earlier comes in useful here.

Look at your life: which areas are shaky or troubled? Consult Chapter 2 for help, if you need to. That chapter is meant to give you a good idea of how the chakra system maps onto the different areas of life. It explains what can happen when each chakra is out of balance. I'll also cover chakra imbalances in this chapter, as well as what you can do about them.

For example, if you feel uncomfortable expressing your feelings in a relationship, your heart chakra might be too constrained. To restore balance, you'll want to do practices to open that chakra specifically.

Or maybe you find yourself being *too* giving and *too* selfless. You may be heedless of your own needs. In that case, finding balance can mean closing the heart chakra somewhat, while working on strengthening other chakras that might be putting you in a weak position—perhaps strengthening your willpower by working on the navel chakra, or your self-expression with the throat chakra.

So the first step is to identify where the imbalances might be occurring. That will take some introspection and thinking, and maybe some trial and error. That's okay. It's a process. It takes time.

Then, once you know the imbalance, you can target specific areas for improvement. There's no one-size-fits-all solution. You just have to get to know yourself a bit, do some reflection, and then get to work on it, which is a learning process in and of itself.

In what follows, I'll explain a bit about what you can do to balance each chakra. I've given more weight to practical steps you can take to change how you conduct your life. That's because you can always find a lot of information elsewhere about different kinds of crystal and herbal healing techniques, various meditations and so on that are supposed to balance your chakras.

These methods have merit, but if you rely on them alone, then you run the risk of just engaging in solipsistic navel-gazing, and then you wonder where the practical benefit is. The practical benefit comes from taking practical measures. There's no shortcut for that. Other healing techniques are useful, but their role is to supplement and support the concrete changes you make in your life. Someone with balanced chakras should be effective and skilled in the way they live their life, so that's what I've chosen to emphasize here.

1. Balancing Muladhara, the Root Chakra

Signs of imbalance in the root chakra can be a failure of survival instincts, a failure to take care of basic needs related to food, shelter, and finances. It can also include addiction and a loss of interest in taking on life's challenges. If you find that, when adversity comes along, you just don't have much fight in you, you probably need to work on *muladhara*.

Alternately, if you're *too* survival-oriented, you might be living in a bunker or off the grid a cabin in the woods with a stash of gold bars hidden under the floorboards. But chances are you have the other problem, because for most of us our modern life cushions us from immediate danger, which dulls our animal instincts.

There are a many techniques you can use to balance muladhara, ranging from the obviously practical to the less obviously so. Here are a few things you can do:

- **Go camping.** Go out into the wilderness alone. Bring only what you need for shelter, cooking, and self-defense. It's even better if the location is pretty remote and there's some danger involved. Why? Because nothing kicks a flagging survival instinct into gear like giving yourself a concrete reminder that you're an animal, too, and the name of the game is survival of the fittest.

- In that vein, you can also **do some death-defying sport** like skydiving or bungee jumping. The specifics don't matter. Just make sure it's thrilling and risky. Again, the idea is to shock your survival instinct into action. But don't sue me if it all goes sideways and you end up in a hospital bed or six feet underground, because this is *inherently risky*. You're just going to have to take responsibility for whatever happens, good or bad.

- Grab a journal and take some time to **write down what will happen if you let your worst habits run amok.** I think you probably already have a good idea of where your weaknesses lie, so be honest with yourself. Brutally honest. Imagine if you gave your laziness, inertia, ennui, and irresponsibility free reign. What would happen?

    Write it down. Fear it. (Fear is not your enemy. It's an indicator that danger might be present, so learn to respect it.) Then resolve never to let that happen. Take any measures necessary to cultivate pro-survival habits.

- **Be more physical.** Do something physical—sports, exercise, dance—to get in touch with your body. Boxing and martial arts are also great, because they're physical, they hone your senses and instincts, and you might get hurt. Ladies, don't shake your heads. This goes for you, too. Risky activity is not just for the guys.

- **Do yoga.** Later in this book I'll give a brief index of yoga positions useful for balancing each of the seven chakras. But for now, suffice it to say that yoga is an amazing way to balance all the chakras in general. Also, it's physical, so it counts as an instance of the the previous method, too.

- Meditate on the color **red.** Visualize it, especially at the base of the spine, in your root chakra. Wear more red. Wear jewelry with red gemstones, such as ruby. This is the color of the root chakra, so focusing on it will help you tune into that frequency.

- **Eat more root vegetables.** Potatoes, onions, carrots, radishes, beets, and so on. Beets are also red. The earthy quality of these foods resonates with the root chakra.

2. Balancing Svadishthana, the Sacral Chakra

Signs of imbalance of *svadishthana* include sexual frustration, an inability to let yourself go when you're having sex, and loss of interest in sex. More generally, loss of creativity and inspiration. Physically this can manifest as various sexual dysfunctions, such as impotence.

It can also be too energized: an excessive sex drive, and even sex addiction, are signs that maybe you need to dial it down.

Here are some things you can do:

- **Make yourself more attractive.** One of the reasons you might be sexually frustrated or losing interest in sex is because others don't find you attractive. If you addressed that and were getting more attention from potential sexual partners—or from your current partner—chances are, your interest in sex would also increase.

    Now, that's a lot easier said than done. How to attract sexual interest is way beyond the scope of this book. But it's not like there's a shortage of literature and advice on this. Still, a few tips: Get into shape. Wear attractive clothing. Be confident and bold, even if you have to fake it.

- If you're having the opposite problem and your sex drive is too high, then **keep higher standards.** I'm not saying you should be a prude, but maybe it's not a good idea too be too breezy about sex, either. It's a serious matter with potentially serious consequences, and it should be treated that way.

- When you sleep with someone, you entangle yourself with them on an energetic level, also. That affects you mentally and emotionally. So exercise some caution and only choose worthy partners who have healthy minds and treat you respectfully.

- Learn to be more comfortable expressing your sexuality through **dance.** Dancing is very physical and sensual, so it's great way to get in tune with the sacral chakra. This will also open you up to more creative energies. Men who are skeptical about this, just consider that dancing is sexy as hell, and anyone you might be sexually interested in will probably find you more attractive just because you can dance well.

- **Kick the porn habit.** The jury's still out on whether porn increases your sex drive or diminishes your motivation to be intimate with actual, real-life humans, but either way, it's not the ideal way to activate your sacral chakra. Working with the chakras should be about decreasing illusion and becoming more attuned to your inner and outer reality. Looking at images on the screen is the opposite of that and just tricks your brain into thinking sexual opportunity is present.

- If you're in a relationship, **keep the romance alive.** Go on romantic dates. Make dinner for your partner and eat it candlelight. Give them a luxurious full-body massage. Let them give you a massage. Tell them what you love about their body. Get in the hot tub together, or take a bubble bath. Don't have a bath tub? Find some place to go skinny dipping at night.

  Don't let routine and boredom kill the passion. Especially if the relationship is not new, you have to work to keep it alive. So sometimes, just try acting young, stupid, and in love.

- Again, **yoga** brings you in touch with your body. And it induces a healthy and balanced flow of energy in the subtle body, which brings your chakras into balance and encourages healthy sexual function and expression. It will also improve your fitness and physique, which makes you more attractive to other people.

- Visualize **orange**, especially in the area of your sacral chakra. Wear orange clothing and orange-colored gemstones like carnelian and citrine. Psychologically, it will attune your mind to the sacral chakra by resonating with its color.

- **Eat sweet, sticky, juicy, tropical fruits.** There's just something inherently sensual about mangoes and pomegranates (compared to, say, turnips or beans) that can awaken the libido.

3. Balancing Manipura, the Navel Chakra

Signs of imbalance can be timidity or fearfulness, low self-esteem, fear of rejection, over-sensitivity to perceived criticism and insults, poor concentration, passivity, and being extremely self-critical. Physically, imbalance can also manifest as digestion problems.

An excess of energy in this chakra can take the form of over-confidence, anger, stubbornness, an overly demanding personality, excessively aggressive behavior, being heedlessly ambitious to the point of ignoring risks and consequences of your actions for others. In other words, headstrong egotism charging forward blindly. It can also manifest as being excessively judgmental and critical of others.

Here are some things you can do:
- If *manipura* is under-active, try **playing competitive games and sports.** Learning to push your advantage against other players in a competitive arena can do wonders for learning the central lesson of this chakra: the ability to assert your personal willpower in life.

- If *manipura* is over-active, on the other hand, you may want to try **engaging in cooperative activities.** This is also part of being a good member of a team. If you think of life as a complex system of nested games, then one of the most important meta-games is to play fairly. What's the object of the meta-game? To play in such a way that the other players will want to play with you in the future.

  This is basically being a good sport, or a pleasant, fair, and likable person. It doesn't mean being a pushover or a weakling. There's a healthy balance to be struck in life, and if you're always steamrolling other people, they won't want to deal with you in the future. That's your loss, not theirs.

- For an overactive navel chakra, try **letting the other person have their way** sometimes. Not all battles need to be won. Just give in sometimes. And try not to be a sore loser about it. The people in your life will appreciate you for knowing how to pick your battles. And if you sacrifice some of your wants for theirs, you'll be surprised how often they're happy to reciprocate by doing nice things for you.

- If you have the opposite problem and act like a doormat, then **stick up for yourself** sometimes. Okay, so that's easier said than done. Maybe you should start small. Stick to matters where the stakes are low.

  You might not be ready to storm your boss's office and ask for a raise. So just choose an easier goal: "I don't really want to eat Chinese tonight. Let's order a pizza instead." You don't have to declare war, but you can at least voice your desires and push for them a bit. That's a pretty good start.

- If you've got your root chakra and sacral chakras in order, then you've got a good foundation for working on *manipura*. So make sure you don't have any more basic issues to work on first. Once you've got that sorted, you'll be in a better position to assert your willpower.

- Don't forget that some **yoga** positions can help here, as we'll cover in a later section. If you want to understand the benefits here, consider how you hold yourself when you're feeling fearful, passive, or unassertive. Your posture is probably not very good, and chances are your head is not held very high. Most people slump their shoulders and slouch.

   Now consider your posture when you feel relaxed, self-assured, and assertive. You're back is probably straight, your shoulders squared, and you're easily able to make eye contact with others.

   This posture communicates confidence and strength of will. It makes you look like an effective person. And, by a kind of feedback loop that happens between our body and mind, you will *feel* more confidence and effective just by holding yourself that way.

- Meditate on **the color yellow** in the navel chakra. Wear bright yellow clothing. Wear gold jewelry and/or yellow gemstones such as yellow topaz or amber.

- Foods that encourage balance in *manipura* include various cereal grains: wheat, flax, rice, and so on. Bread and pasta resonate with this chakra. Also try adding ginger and turmeric to your food. They promote healthy digestion and healthy functioning of the navel chakra.

4. Balancing Anahata, the Heart Chakra

Imbalance in the heart chakra can manifest as inability to express emotions to others, especially feelings of love and appreciation, but also a failure to express disappointment, sadness, and hurt feelings. You don't need to wear your heart on your sleeve, but it's good if you can share your heart's feelings with the people who are closest to you.

Physical symptoms can include irregular heart rate and arrhythmia, chest pains, even heart attack. Of course, if you're experiencing any of these symptoms, they're very serious. So you should definitely see a doctor about them, and only after that work on balancing the chakra.

An over-active heart chakra takes the form of an overabundance of stormy emotions—excessive sadness, grief, despair, feelings of betrayal and hurt, anger, emotional neediness, and so on. If such emotions sweep through you uncontrollably, making you like a ship out at sea, battered and tossed by stormy winds, then you need to work on the heart chakra.

Anger in the case of an overactive heart chakra is different from an overactive navel chakra. If *manipura* is overactive, anger is the go-to emotional reaction whenever you face frustration or resistance. If *anahata* is overactive, anger is just one emotion in a chaotic flux.

There are many things you can do about an imbalance in the heart chakra:

- If you think your heart chakra is underactive, then right now **pick up the phone and call someone you love**. It could be your mother or father, another relative, a significant other, or a friend. It doesn't matter. Pick someone who you never really communicate with emotionally but who matters to you in your heart. Tell them what they mean to you and how much you appreciate them.

  You don't have to use the L-word if you'd prefer not to. It's not so much which words you use as the meaning: that you care about that person, that they matter to you and you appreciate what they bring to your life.

- If, on the other hand, your life is characterized by emotional turbulence, you will want to step back and take a look at the cause of it.

- Don't leap to the conclusion that the problem is with you. It could be that you have allowed someone into your heart who is not being very kind to you. Does your emotional chaos come from someone else's drama and manipulations? If so, take whatever steps you need to take to **distance yourself from the person who is causing you distress**—cleanly, gently, without hurting or blaming them, but also with a firm resolve and confidence that you have to take your own emotional wellbeing first.

- If the source does not lie with another person, then a solution is more difficult. It could be your emotions are turbulent because anxieties and fears stemming from past traumas.

That's worth considering, but you don't have to keep revisiting painful episodes from the past. **Mindfulness meditation** is a good way to get some critical distance from your emotions.

The point of mindfulness is not to perform an emotional amputation. The point is to get in touch with the background, the space, in which emotions are occurring. The energy of emotions is very vivid and raw, but they occur in a changeless space of naked awareness. Abide in the awareness rather than in the constant movement of emotional energy. When you learn to rest in that intrinsic openness, emotional turbulence will subside on its own.

- To that end, you might want to **join a meditation course**. Zen meditation is a very good option for people who suffer from excessive emotions and thoughts, because it's very disciplined and doesn't offer any room for distractions and entertainment. If you can find a local Zen center where you can get meditation instruction and sit *zazen*, you will make great strides to fostering a greater sense of inner peace and emotional calm.

  Insight meditation or *vipassana* is also another very powerful form of meditation for cultivating a peaceful, accurate, and spacious mind. There's also a lot of scientific research on insight meditation and other kinds of mindfulness meditation that proves its effectiveness for treating depression and anxiety.

- Again, **yoga** is very good for encouraging emotional balance. You will know this if you've ever had a really good, healing yoga session. You just *feel* better, physically and emotionally. For the heart chakra as with all chakras, there are specific poses you can do to target it for balancing and healing.

- Meditate on **the color green**, especially green light in the center of your chest. Wear green clothing and/or green jewelry, such as emerald, jade, or green quartz.
- Surround yourself with greenery by **visiting the park or a botanical garden**, or going on a hike. The human mind loves plants and feels happier and at ease amongst trees, grass, and flowers.
- **Do some gardening** or keep potted plants and take care of them. Aside from the previous point about greenery, gardening helps you get in touch with the caring side of yourself, because you have to take responsibility for the growth and health of another living thing. It's a good way to develop your nurturing side without raising a kid or having to clean up poop.
- Eat **leafy green vegetables**—spinach, kale, broccoli, and so on. Herbal teas, especially tulsi, are also healing for the heart chakra.

5. Balancing Vishuddha, the Throat Chakra

The lower four chakras are connected with the vital, worldly needs people have, which build on top of one another: survival, reproduction, will, and love. Love is the nexus between the higher and lower priorities of human life. It is the pivot between the worldly and spiritual planes of our existence. You have to take care of these priorities before you can work on the spiritual levels.

Imbalance in *vishuddha* can take the form of an inability or failure to express yourself, poor verbal communication, inarticulate speech. If what you say is constantly being misunderstood by others, it might be because you're not saying it well. That is the sign of an underdeveloped throat chakra.

Other signs of imbalance include frequent lying, dissembling, or any dishonest speech. Insincere speech, gossip, and meaningless chatter can also indicate an overactive throat chakra. Maybe you're too forceful in the way you express your opinions—others find you opinionated and wish you would keep quiet sometimes.

Physically, the feeling of a "lump in your throat" is a symptom that this chakra is receiving more energy than it can handle. Constant problems connected with the throat—sore throat, laryngitis, tonsilitis, etc. can be connected to an imbalance in *vishuddha*.

Here's what you can do:

- **Keep a journal or diary.** Just write more. Writing is also a form of self-expression, and if you can learn to write more articulately, you can learn to speak more articulately, as well.
- **Learn another language.** It's hard to do, but it definitely increases your verbal abilities. It also expands your mind: language influences how we think, and if we speak a different language, we will also come to think differently. Or at least we will expand the scope of our thinking. It's a good mental challenge.
- The throat chakra is connected not just with verbal speech, but with the literary arts, singing, and music. Any kind of **learning** will develop this chakra. **Taking up a musical instrument** or singing lessons will also bring an under-active throat chakra into balance. Even if you just sing in the shower, that's pretty good, too. Just sing your heart out. Don't be shy.

- **Be careful what you say.** Learn to practice mindfulness in speech. If you pay attention to how you feel emotionally and physically when you speak, you'll quickly find that there's a big difference between honest and dishonest speech. If you speak dishonestly or insincerely and too carelessly, you will have a bad feeling. It will register physiologically, also.

  If you speak true words that are helpful to others and meaningful, it will strengthen you emotionally and physically. You will become a more trustworthy and respected person. People will listen to you, heed your advice, and give importance to your words. You'll have a gravitas that cannot be ignored.

- Visualize a **light-blue**, healing light in your throat. Wear sky-blue clothes. Gaze at the bright blue sky on a cloudless day and let your sense of awareness expand with it. Wear blue-colored gemstones such as sapphire or turquoise.

- Drinking more water, juice, and other liquids helps bring healing and balance to this chakra. Sour fruits like lemon and kiwi also help. More salt intake also benefits the throat chakra.

6. Balancing Ajña, the Third Eye Chakra

Signs of imbalance in *ajña* might be an underdeveloped spiritual side. That might include lack of imagination or excessive cynicism and skepticism about spirituality (a moderate amount of skepticism is healthy). Maybe you also lack common sense, intelligence, or a sharp intuition about things.

An overactive *ajña* might involve getting lost in daydreams and fantasies. Or it could mean a completely unrealistic, fantastical "spirituality" that's disconnected from the concrete realities of daily life. You might imagine you see all sorts of visions in meditation, for example, when you're really just deluding yourself.

Physical symptoms can include headaches and various brain problems.

Here's what you can do:

- If your third eye chakra is under-active, then try to **remember your dreams**. Write them down when you first wake up in the morning. Consider their meaning.
- If it helps, learn more about dream interpretation, such as **Jungian depth psychology**. There's a deeper symbolic meaning to dreams and myths, and learning to speak this language will not only give you a deeper appreciation for life's spiritual side, but it will also allow you to consult the guidance of your innermost self by understanding the language of symbols that it speaks.
- **Pay attention to coincidences.** Coincidences can be meaningful. Meaningful coincidences are called *synchronicities*. Don't go overboard with this, or you could end up in a fantasy world of your own devising. Don't take synchronicities 100% seriously. Instead, take them somewhere in the range of 50-90% seriously, and only look to them for guidance if they resonate with you on a deep level of truth.
- If you have the opposite problem and are adrift in an unreal, false "spirituality" of fantasy, then that's probably because you're using spirituality to escape from more concrete problems in your worldly existence. So **work on your lower chakras**. There's something there that you're avoiding. Pay attention to it.

- **Don't go off the deep-end with drugs**, especially drugs that have a dreamlike effect. You know which ones I'm talking about. Whatever you enjoy, enjoy it in moderation.

- Meditate on an **indigo-colored light** at the center of your brow. Imagine it healing you and infusing you with a divine insight and sharper, more penetrating perception.

7. Balancing Sahasrara, the Crown Chakra

Almost no one has balanced this chakra, because it's closed for almost everyone. *Sahasrara* is a secret that conceals itself. This is your direct link to the Divine, to the absolute source of being-as-such. Occasionally it might open spontaneously in a moment of spiritual ecstasy and revelation. But to have the floodgates open all the time would be intolerable for most people unless all the other six chakras were very well balanced and healthy, with a balanced flow of energy between them.

If you have no sense of connection with the divine, with your life's purpose, no sense of meaning or ultimate identity, that suggests that your connection with this chakra is completely shut down.

Here are some first steps you can take to make a connection to your higher self:

- One way to connect to this chakra is to do more spiritual activities such as **meditation and prayer.** Here the goal of meditation is a bit different. It's not about finding emotional balance or peace. It's more about slowly undoing the games of ego. *Sahasrara* transcends ego and limited, mundane ego identity. You are surrendering the limited, worldly ego to a higher plane of being. So activating this chakra is the endgame of spiritual practice. It's not something you can expect to achieve right now, but you can start working towards it.

- If you're feeling adrift, without meaning, and want to connect to your sense of higher purpose, then read about the **lives of great spiritual masters**. Contemplate their example: the selfless, heroic way they conducted their lives with gentleness and compassion, how they treated others, how they carried themselves. This will give you a sense of what human life is when lived at its level of highest purpose.

- The **color white** contains all the colors in the visible spectrum, while at the same time it suggests a purity, untouched by the dirt of the world. Meditate on a bright white light at your crown, which refracts into a rainbow prism of a thousand colors at the edges. Imagine that this light fills you with a sense of higher purpose beyond your personal concerns and connects you with a divine consciousness.

- Wear more white clothing. Wear white or transparent gemstones such as diamond or clear quartz.

Chapter 4: Working with the Chakras

At this point, you are probably getting a sense of the magnitude of the subject. The subtle body, and the yogic systems that operate on it, are extremely complex topics. As I mentioned before, although the seven-chakra system is the most popular in modern times, there are many other systems as well. There are also many systems of practice for the chakras, both ancient and modern.

The fact of the matter is, there is no quick and dirty way of opening the chakras. And if there were, it would be extremely inadvisable for a beginner to attempt such a thing. The untrained person's chakras are not very functional. They mostly lie dormant, although they may stir from time to time. To suddenly throw open the doors to their operation would invite all sorts of dangers.

Unfortunately, people who prematurely open their chakras, whether accidentally or on purpose, can end up institutionalized. They can suffer from hallucinations, disassociation, delusions, paranoia, and so on. It is much better to go with a gradual program of cleansing and balancing them as a preparation to one day opening them, should you ever choose to do so. The previous chapter gave you some practical tips on how to do that.

Still, I'd like to give a rough overview of what such a path would look like. This is an aerial view, a broad outline, intended only to give a general idea of the shape of things. We'll go also over some beginning practices for starting to make contact with the energies of the chakras and giving them a bit of a tune-up. These practices are meant as entry points for beginners. If you find that this path feels right for you, you should seek out a teacher and consult the more advanced literature on the topic.

Kundalini

We have talked a bit about kundalini already, and how it relates to the whole system of the subtle body and the goal of yogic practice. Properly covering kundalini would require at least another book, but we'll say a few more words about it here.

A kundalini awakening refers to the arousal of the dormant energy that lies coiled at the *muladhara* chakra at the base of the spine. There are two ways that this energy can awaken: intentionally, as a result of practices meant to awaken it and raise it up, and unintentionally, in sensitive individuals who respond to some trigger.

While spontaneous eruptions of kundalini are known to occur prematurely and unintentionally, they are somewhat unusual and definitely undesirable. When this happens, the suddenly aroused energy of kundalini can blast upwards quite forcefully. I have already mentioned some of the possible fallout of chakras prematurely opening.

Hatha Yoga

The physical body is purified and trained through the practice of hatha yoga, which is more or less the kind of dynamic, physical yoga now famous all over the world. It involves the union of bodily movement and meditative concentration. This prepares the body for sitting for long periods in order to practice pranayama, or breath control. But the various positions or asanas of hatha yoga themselves help purify the chakras and bring them into balance. The following is a list of asanas useful for working with the chakras:

1. *Muladhara*: siddhasana, tadasana, tiryaka tadasana, marjari asana
2. *Svadishthana*: siddhasana, ustrasana, padahastasana, bhujangasana, paschimottasana
3. *Manipura*: advasana, makarasana, tiryaka tadasana, ashtanga namaskara, bhujangasana, dhanurasana, setu asana, halasana
4. *Anahata*: bhujangasana, dhanurasana
5. *Vishudda*: ustrasana, hasta utthanasana, parvatasana, bhujangasana, dhanurasana, halasana
6. *Ajña*: shavasana, advasana, tadasana, ashva sanchalanasana, bhujangasana

Finally, the classic position for seated meditation, the lotus position or padmasana, calms the subtle energies and directs their flow upward from the root chakra to the crown chakra.

All of these asanas can be found in my other book, The Yoga Beginner's Bible. **(http://a.co/1abQ2xD)**

Pranayama

Pranayama is often translated "breath control." Here the word *prana* does not mean breath, precisely, but the subtle energy that is connected with the breath. Pranayama works directly with this energy by manipulating the breath through a number of different exercises involving inhalation, exhalation, and internal and external retention of the breath. These influence the flow of prana through the channels of the subtle body.

There are many pranayama practices, but one of the simplest ones to encourage the health of the chakras is called *anuloma viloma pranayama*, or alternate nostril breathing. It is relatively safe for beginners to practice:

- Begin by sitting cross legged, with your back straight. Lotus position (*padmasana*) and the masters' pose (*siddhasana*) are ideal positions, but if they are too strenuous for you, sit in the more comfortable position of *sukhasana*. All of these positions are explained in my yoga book, The Yoga Beginner's Bible.
- Rest your left hand on your knee.
- Fold the index and middle fingers of your right hand. Your thumb and ring and pinky fingers should be extended.
- Close your eyes and breathe slowly and gently for ten breaths. Just relax and remain mindful of the breath.
- Press your right thumb gently against your right nostril to close it. Breathe in slowly through the left nostril. Breathe in fully, with your entire diaphragm and chest.
- Now release the right nostril and close the left nostril with your ring finger. Breathe out slowly through your right nostril, completely expelling all air from your lungs.
- Without moving your fingers, keep your left nostril closed, and breathe in fully through the right nostril.
- Again close the right nostril with the right thumb and slowly breathe out through the left nostril, emptying the lungs.
- This completes one round. Do seven rounds a day, preferably in the early morning when your mind is clear of thoughts, or in the evening just after sunset. Don't practice alternate nostril breathing directly during sunrise or sunset.
- After completing seven rounds, rest your right hand on your knee and simply relax your attention. Let the

breath rise and fall naturally, without conscious interference. Rest in the open field of awareness without getting distracted by the train of thoughts or concentrating on anything in particular.

There are more advanced forms of alternate nostril breathing that involve adjusting the ratio of the duration of inhalation and exhalation, but for starters, this simple version is an excellent way to soothe the energy in the body. Alternate nostril breathing balances the flow of energy in the left and right channels, *ida* and *pingala*. This brings about a feeling of balance, centeredness, and peace of mind. It purifies the two channels and encourages good health by inducing the flow of energy to the body's organs. By balancing the left and right channels, it stimulates the flow of energy in the central channel, which heals the chakras and causes them to come into balance.

There are many other pranayama practices, such as breath of fire (agni prasana), but they are beyond the scope of this book. Pranayama traditionally comes after a period of training the body through yoga positions and should be practiced in alongside asanas. Like all of the practices mentioned in this book, it is best performed under the guidance of a qualified and experienced teacher, who can give you personal instruction and adjust the methods according to your particular needs.

* * *

Before we jump into a description of the next exercise, let's talk a bit about the notion of samskaras. *Samskara* can be translated as formation or conditioning. All negative experiences from the past, from minor ones to major traumas, create negative samskaras in the body-mind. They may make us feel more vulnerable or defensive. They condition our reactions to certain stimuli. These samskaras are left as impressions on the chakras, and they modify that chakra's energy in unhealthy ways.

As an extreme example, a soldier returning from war with PTSD might have very strong samskaras imprinted on his root and heart chakras. These samskaras might take the form of a nagging feeling of danger stored in the root chakra, which sometimes erupts into a full-blown episode when he feels particularly unsafe. Or it may be a shutdown of the energy of the heart chakra, as a result of guilt over the extreme violence of wartime.

Before any truly spiritual work can begin, it is necessary to work on these samskaras by gently healing and balancing the chakras. If you try to jump into more advanced practice too soon, a sudden awakening of kundalini energy could blast through the chakras, unleashing all these impressions at once and triggering a psychotic break. So the first steps should involve establishing a secure foundation by leading a healthy lifestyle, training the body through yoga, and balancing its energies through the more gentle pranayama practices. We can also begin to work on the chakras in a gentle way through visualization and mantra.

Visualization

- Begin by finding a comfortable position in a place where you will not be disturbed for the duration of the meditation. A seated position is best, with legs crossed. Keep your back straight.

- Close your eyes and feel the weight of your body on the floor or the cushion. Just rest your attention on the heft of the body, the weight of your limbs, the feeling of the ground or floor beneath you. Allow your mind to rest there for a few moments, aware of the solid quality of the earth beneath you.

- Take five deep breaths. Just draw the breath in, fill your lungs, and let it out with a sigh. With each outbreath, you go into a deeper and deeper relaxation. Then let the breath relax naturally, and just place your attention on the breath itself. Allow yourself to feel the breath fully. There is a cooling sensation as it enters your nostrils. Your chest rises and falls with the breath. Each breath carries life-giving oxygen into your body, as well as the rejuvenating energy of prana, the pulse of the universe.

- Relinquish your attention and relax it completely, then turn your mind inwards to your subtle body. Start by focusing your attention on the root chakra at the base of the spine. This is in the area of the perineum, near the anus. Simply rest your awareness there and feel any energy or sensation you might have in this region. Appreciate the earthy, grounding quality of this chakra.

- Turn your mind to the meaning of *muladhara* for a sense of security and survival. Consider the meaning of this in your life, how it might relate to your financial or living situation. Imagine what you would do differently if this chakra were optimally balanced.

- In your mind's eye, imagine a four-petaled, red flower made of light where the root chakra is located. Feel its energy at the base of the spine. Visualize the light from the chakra growing brighter and clearer, purifying anything that might be obscuring it and soothing any physical or emotional pain you might have at this level.
- Now rest your awareness slightly above the root chakra, at the sacrum behind the genitals. Allow yourself to feel the energy of the sacral chakra.
- Contemplate the meaning of *svadishthana*, which is connected to sexuality, desire, and passion. Relate it to your own life, your own sexuality and sensuality. It doesn't have to be sexuality—it can be any sensual pleasure that gives you enjoyment, such as good food. Are you overindulgent? Or repressed? Think about how you would live if you had an optimal relationship to your own passions and sensory desires.
- Imagine a six-petaled lotus made of orange light. Feel its pulsing energy. Imagine that the light becomes more intense. It doesn't necessarily radiate, but the brightness turns up. Its flowing, watery quality washes away any negativity and pain, leaving the chakra clean and bright.
- Move your attention up to the navel chakra, which is located behind the navel region somewhere in the belly. Just rest the mind there and feel its energy. Reflect on the meaning of *manipura* in your life just as you did with the previous two chakras. Then imagine a ten-petaled lotus flower of yellow light. Turn up the light, making it brighter and clearer. Imagine that its fiery energy warms your abdomen and burns away any obstructions or imbalances in your willpower, as well as any digestive problems you might have.

- Direct your attention to the center of your chest, the heart chakra. Feel the quiet, warm and tender energy of *anahata* resting gently in your chest. Reflect on *anahata* in a personal manner as before. Then imagine that there is a twelve-petaled lotus of green light at the location of this chakra. Slowly the light gets brighter and clearer. Its windy energy blows away the clouds that obscure your sense of affection and love for others, any negativities or defense mechanisms that block your tenderheartedness. This wind clears away the clouds and cools any heartache or sadness you might feel, leaving you with a pervasive sense of gentleness and kindness.

- Move your attention to your throat chakra. Feel any energy located in this area, any tension or relaxation—just feel the energy and notice it without trying to modify it. Reflect on the meaning of the *vishuddha* chakra in your life, for your own use of speech—is your speech constructive and well-considered? Do you have any inhibitions about expressing yourself? Imagine a lotus of sixteen petals. It's made of sky-blue light. The light slowly grows brighter and clearer. Any sense of dullness dissolves into its spacious quality, and you feel a sense of openness and relaxation in the throat.

- Then move your attention to the third eye chakra behind your forehead. Feel the energy of this chakra as it is now. Look at the quality of your thoughts and your mind. Is your mind calm or overactive? Clear or dull? Do you imagine things to be true that are not true? Reflect on the meaning of *ajña*, your mind, the command center. Then imagine a two-petaled lotus of deep indigo light sits in the location of this chakra. Its light slowly becomes brighter and more intense. The sharpness and penetrating clarity of its energy dispel any confusion and pierce the rigidity of clinging to beliefs. Its light breaks through illusions, fantasies, delusions, and paranoia.

- Slowly move your awareness down to your throat chakra again, then to your heart chakra, and so on, down to root chakra. You don't need to visualize anything this time. Just linger briefly on each chakra and feel its energy. Imagine that you feel a sense of balance and peace in each chakra. When you reach the root chakra, once again feel the weight of your body. Allow your mind to return from the subtle body to the gross, physical body.

- When you're ready, open your eyes and look around you. Don't get up just yet. Just sit for a moment, letting your consciousness return to its normal waking state.

That's it. Notice that this meditation leaves out any mention of the crown chakra. That's on purpose. Unfolding the energy of the crown chakra requires long and patient work on the lower chakras. Any premature attempt to tap into its energy could lead to disaster.

Notice also that this meditation involves, in the end, *returning* to the root chakra and the body. It begins and ends with grounding yourself in an awareness of physicality. This is important, because it keeps you in touch with the solidity of everyday life. Although with the chakras, your spirituality can soar to celestial heights, it's still important to keep your feet firmly planted on the ground.

Sounding the Seed Syllables

Remember in the section on the chakras, how each chakra has an associated mantra or seed syllable? In this section we'll touch on what that's all about.

The most famous mantra is the simple sound *Om* or *Aum*, the uncreated, primordial sound of the cosmos that expresses absolute reality. It is in and sounds through all things, if you can tune into its frequency. Likewise, the ancient yogic conception of reality has it that certain vocal sounds are tuned into certain levels of experience. So each of the chakras has its own sound, and by reciting or intoning its seed syllable, you can connect to its energy.

One way of doing this is just to sit in meditation, close your eyes, and intone the appropriate seed syllable of whichever chakra you want to work with. In this kind of practice, you just rest your attention on the sound itself. Allow your mind to merge with the sound of the mantra.

You can also recite the seed syllables in conjunction with the previous meditation. Once you are used to the visualization process, intone the appropriate seed syllable while you imagine the form and color of the lotus of that chakra. Feel the vibration of the sound in your body, moving through the appropriate chakra. You can search for the syllables on Youtube if you're unsure of their pronunciation.

For convenient reference, here is a list of the chakras with their associated sounds. All of them rhyme except the last one, *Om*:

1. Muladhara: *Lam* (pronounced "lum," rhymes with "some")
2. Svadishthana: *Vam*

3. Manipura: *Ram*
4. Anahata: *Yam*
5. Vishuddha: *Ham*
6. Ajña: *Om*

Essential Oils for the Chakras

There are innumerable ways to balance the chakras. As I mentioned earlier, some of them are supplementary methods. Using essential oils and incenses won't fix any serious problems, but it can support the other kinds of work you do to balance the chakras.

One way is through aromatherapy. You can burn incense or heat essential oils to promote healthy functioning of the chakras.

1. For the root chakra, patchouli, vetiver, benzoin, and angelica are helpful.
2. For the sacral chakra, try ylang-ylang, jasmine, neroli, and rose.
3. For the navel chakra, there are juniper, rosemary, and peppermint, hyssop, and cardamom.
4. For the heart chakra, try using geranium, bergamot, mandarine, rosewood, and melissa.
5. For the throat chakra, blue chamomile, lemongrass, and cypress are restorative.
6. For the third eye chakra, peppermint, spruce, juniper, and thyme are excellent.

For the crown chakra, use frankincense, sandalwood, myrrh, lavender, or St. John's Wort.

Chapter 5: Healing the Chakras

In previous chapters, we went over some of the ways you can balance the chakras. We covered some very hands-on, practical things you can do to get a working knowledge of how the chakras relate to your life. Most of the material had to do with everyday activity and getting out into the world.

Then we discussed a basic outline for working with the chakras, to get them open and humming.

But some of us may not be ready for such an approach. Those who have experienced trauma might find that they carry their wounds with them. When an extreme or emotionally shocking event happens to us, then it can blow out the fuse of the chakras. A chakra gets a surge of energy it's not prepared to receive and short-circuits.

The traumas and memories of the past leave their imprint on the chakras, and the chakra shuts down, getting blocked completely. It's as if the chakra throws up a defense shield or protective barrier around itself to prevent further injury—like a hard, impenetrable shell.

That defense shield can be very hard to break through. If you've experienced trauma connected to the root chakra, for example, it will be too frightening to jump into activities that cause your survival instinct to kick in. You run the danger instead of shutting down and reliving the trauma, which could only serve to harden the protective shell around that chakra.

In that case, it's better to take an easy-going tack and work towards healing the chakra slowly. Healing the wounded chakras involves soothing them, progressively loosening that hard shell it until it slowly begins to yield and become pliable.

Figuring Out the Problem

The first thing you'll want to do when healing the chakras is to identify which chakra, or chakras, you need to work on. That means you have to think about your problem.

It's not always clear which problem has to do with which chakra. For example, say you have crippling shyness and social anxiety. It has reached an extreme point where it's interfering with your life—your social life, no doubt, maybe also your career. Which chakra does that correspond to?

- First consider the **context**. When does it come up? If you start to panic and get tense inside when it comes to talking to someone of the opposite sex (or anyone you might be sexually interested in), then the problem is probably connected with your sacral chakra, which governs sexuality.

  Or maybe you've been giving your time and energy to your work, creating value for your company. But it freaks you out too much to ask your boss for a raise that you desperately deserve. Then the problem has to do with assertion and willpower—connected to the navel chakra.

  Maybe you don't feel confident to express yourself effectively. You want to communicate but can't find the right words. Then the problem might have to do with the throat chakra.

- Also **notice what kinds of thoughts you have** when your problem comes up. Do you get preoccupied with fear about your money situation, or start to panic when you think about finances? You might want to work on healing your root chakra.

When you are getting closer to someone emotionally, do you start to have doubts and suspicions about them? If you're being as objective as possible, are those doubts rooted in reality? If you're being very suspicious and mistrustful of the people close to you for no reason, then you'll want to consider healing work on the heart chakra.

So pay attention to your state of mind and what kind of thoughts are happening in your head. It will help you figure out the nature of the problems that are troubling you.

- **Notice emotions and feelings** that come up as well. How do you feel when someone close to you shows their love or affection? Do you feel the same emotions in your own heart? Do you feel afraid or uncomfortable? Or apathetic? If something feels off, you'll want to work on your heart chakra.

    How do you feel when the topic of spirituality comes up? Maybe you have your own spiritual beliefs sorted out. But maybe not. Do you feel cynical or angry when people express a spiritual point of view? Or maybe uncomfortable? Do you feel a compulsion to change other people's beliefs when they're different from yours? These could be signs that the crown chakra needs work.

- **Pay attention to where emotions register in your body.** When your problem comes up, you probably feel a rush of energy somewhere in your body. It could be a sinking feeling in your gut. Maybe it's a lump in your throat. Or it could be a feeling in the area of your heart. Wherever the energy is active in your body, these physiological sensations are clues about which chakra is in play.

Those are some preliminary steps you'll want to take to diagnose the problem. So set aside some time to slow down and think about the points above. Rest, maybe do some meditation, then turn your attention inward and look at yourself. Don't flinch from what you see, but investigate honestly and fearlessly.

You'll also want to continue your chakra diagnostics as you go through the following meditations. I've highlighted some points when you'll want to pay careful attention.

In general, it's always a good idea to keep 10-20% percent of your awareness on your thoughts, feelings, physiological sensations. Just be aware of anything that is happening in your body or mind. That will help you do some fine-tuning and make on-the-fly adjustments wherever appropriate.

A Meditation to Heal the Wounded Chakras

1. Find a comfortable place, such as a bed or a sofa, where you will not be disturbed.
2. Lie on your back and close your eyes. You may prefer to bend your knees and keep your feet flat on the ground.
3. Relax your body completely, starting with the the muscles in your head and face, moving down to your neck, shoulders, then your arms. Then relax your upper back and chest. Following that, your lower back and abdomen. Then progressively relax your groin, legs, and feet.
4. Breathing slowly, place your attention on the breath. Count from 1 to 7, resting your mind on the inbreath and outbreath each time. When you reach 7, start again at 1. Do this several times, until your mind relaxes into an expansive and meditative state.

If your mind wanders from the breath, that's no problem. Just gently return to your attention to your breathing, letting your mind rest on the gentle rise and fall of the breath.

You might have some other meditation technique for getting into that meditative zone of restfulness and healing. If you prefer to use it at this point, that's no problem. The idea is just to make your awareness expansive and meditative. So use whatever works for you.

5. Now bring to mind the wound that pains you—whatever inner wound it is you need to heal. Don't dwell on it or think about it so much, like picking at a scab with your mind. Simply feel the pain and the emotion that goes with it.

    Get a sense of what it is like and how it feels, without accepting or rejecting it as good or bad. Sometimes just allowing yourself to experience pain this way can jump start the healing process.

6. Once you've allowed yourself to feel your pain directly, without judgment, turn your attention to the manifestation of energy in the body: Where in the body do you feel any sensations connected with the emotion? Is the energy moving or staying in one place? Is it warm or cold? Tense? What other felt qualities does it have?

7. Feeling the energy in the body can help you locate the chakra you need to heal, as well as any peripheral areas connected to that wound. Try to feel, physiologically and energetically, the knot, tension, or defensive shell that has built up around the chakra. Probe it gently with your mind, to get a sense of how hard or soft it is, firm or yielding, and so on.

8. Envision your higher power in the space above you. If you are religious, you may want to envision a figure from your religion. You can envision your holy guardian angel or someone else. If you prefer, you can visualize your higher power in another way—as a sphere of white light, for example. If you're not religious, think of it as your inmost self in visible shape.

9. From your higher power comes a beam of light that touches your wounded chakra. The color of the light is the same as the color of the chakra. If you are healing your heart chakra, the light will be green. If it's the sacral chakra, the light will be orange, and so on.

10. Imagine the light slowly penetrating the chakra. If the energy of the chakra is hot, the light will have a refreshing cooling effect. If the energy of the chakra is cold, the light gently warms it. Slowly it begins to dissolve the shell surrounding the chakra. Slowly it melts the energetic knots that bind and stifle the energy of that chakra. It also gently heals any wounds and melts away the physical and emotional pain.

    All pain and negativity exit the body like a black ooze and spill onto the ground, sinking into the earth. Allow yourself to really feel the pain and woundedness slowly heal and ebb away. It's like you were having a bad dream, and now you're waking up.

    Let the light take its time to perform its healing work. There's no need to rush this part of the meditation— allow enough time for the healing to do a thorough job.

11. Once you feel healed, silently give thanks to your higher power for healing you. You might want to say a prayer of thanks in your mind, or you can silently join your palms in front of you as a sign of respect.

12. Just rest in the feeling of relief, happiness, love—or whatever positive emotion you are feeling. Don't try to maintain or prolong the feeling, particularly. Just let it be, just allow your mind to relax in that state. Remain there for as long as you like, just enjoying the soothing goodness of that positive state.

13. After some time, your mind will naturally want to return to the external world again. When it begins to do so, open your eyes. Continue to lie down for two or three minutes, just breathing and remaining aware of the environment around you—the space between objects, the quality of light.

14. When you're ready, rise up from your reclining position. Carry out your everyday activities slowly and easily.

    I say to do things slowly because the newly healed chakra is still sensitive, so you will want to avoid bringing too much energy into your system too quickly. It's best to do simple, grounding tasks—washing the dishes, taking a bath, and so on. Avoid the screens; laptops and phones will bring too much energy into the head. It's better to keep the energy grounded.

Canal Locks

The previous meditation exercise was kind of a spot treatment for chakra healing. It focuses on one problematic area to dissolve acute trauma to the chakras. But what if you're looking for a more holistic approach that works on all seven chakras?

The following meditation is a good way to gently work on healing each chakra one by one, starting from the root chakra and working all the way up to the crown.

One of its main advantages is that it isolates the circuits between the chakras, so the energy of prana is not free to move between the root and crown. This reduces the risk of kundalini awakening before you're ready for it. If your chakras are in need of this kind of healing, you don't want to open a continuous circuit from bottom to top. That would blow out your whole system. So this meditation isolates the prana in each circuit before opening the next one.

Think of it as a series of canal locks, as in the Panama Canal. As one lock opens, the other closes behind it. That allows the energy to move incrementally, one circuit at a time. Don't worry, the analogy will make sense in a moment when we get into the details of the meditation.

1. Lie down as before, on your back with your knees bent and together, feet flat on the floor.
2. Relax your body, starting from the crown of your head and working your way down through the muscles in your face and jaw, your neck, shoulders, upper back, chest, arms, torso, groin, legs, and feet. Properly feel the tension in each area ease and dissolve away.
3. Using mindfulness of the breath or any other preferred meditation technique, relax into a state of mental calm, where your awareness is restful but clear and alert. This is the "sweet spot" of meditative calm that allows healing to take place.
4. Breathe in deeply to your perineum or root chakra like a bellows, filling the spot with prana. Breathe out again, and imagine any negative energy leaving through your nostrils.

    As you do so, squeeze the muscles in your groin to stimulate the root chakra. Again breathe the energy into and out from your root chakra, until you feel that it is clear and any negativity is expelled. Do this several times. On each exhalation, intone the syllable *lam* (pronounced "lum")—the mantra of the root chakra— letting it resonate and vibrate in the chakra.

5. On your next inhalation, imagine that your in-breath pulls the energy up from the root chakra into the sacral chakra. Hold the breath for just a second or two, keeping the energy in the sacral chakra and allowing it to suffuse the chakra. Then, as you breathe out, the energy circulates back down towards the root chakra.

   Keep cycling the energy between the root chakra and sacral chakra several times. This establishes a circuit between the two chakras, as if electricity is cycling through them. As you exhale, intone the syllable *vam*, the mantra of the sacral chakra, and feel it vibrate through that chakra.

   Keep repeating this until the energy starts to move effortlessly by itself and dissolves any wounds or scars in the chakras.

6. Then, on the next inbreath, pull the prana up from the root chakra and into the solar plexus chakra. Again hold the breath for a moment, allowing it to penetrate and loosen the chakra. Then breathe out, bringing the prana back to the root chakra. Repeat the cycle several times until it feels natural.

   Then inhale the prana into the solar plexus and close the root chakra to reduce the circuit, so that the energy is moving between the sacral chakra and the solar plexus chakra. Keep repeating that circuit, bring prana up with the inbreath and down with the outbreath. Do that until the energy is circulating quite easily without effort. On each exhalation, intone the syllable *ram*, the mantra of the solar plexus chakra.

7. Now increase the circuit again, pulling the energy from the sacral chakra into the heart chakra with your inhalation. Allow it to circulate among the three chakras for some time. Then, on the last inbreath, hold it in the heart chakra and close the sacral chakra.

   Exhale and bring the energy into the solar plexus. Continue to circulate it between the heart chakra and solar plexus. On each exhalation, intone the syllable *yam* of the heart chakra.

8. Then again enlarge the circuit, bringing the energy up into the throat chakra on the inhalation. Let it circulate from the throat chakra to the solar plexus several times, then reduce the circuit again, so that the energy circulates between the throat chakra and heart chakra. Intone the syllable *ham* of the throat chakra.

9. Next, pull the energy from the heart chakra to the third eye. Circulate it several times. Then close the heart chakra and let it cycle between the third eye and throat chakra until it feels natural and effortless. On exhaling, intone *om*, the mantra of the third eye chakra.

10. Then enlarge the circuit so the energy moves between the throat chakra and the crown chakra. Allow it to cycle between them several times, then close the throat chakra and reduce the circuit to the third eye chakra and crown chakras. Continue breathing as before, pulling the energy up when you inhale and back down when you exhale.

11. This next part is a crucial step, which you shouldn't skip over. Once the energy has circulated between your third eye and crown chakras, again enlarge the circuit by opening the throat chakra again. Then reduce the circuit to the throat chakra and third eye.

12. Just as you stepped up the ladder of the chakras, progressively increasing and reducing each circuit, now you step down, until the energy is once more circulating between the sacral chakra and root chakra.

13. Finally close the chakra, and breathe energy in and out of the root chakra several times. As you went up and down the scale of the seven chakras, the prana may have picked up some negativity on its journey. Now that you're back to the level of the root chakra, you can expel it. Just breathe it out and imagine that it leaves your body completely, leaving your subtle energy system clean and clear.

14. Continuing lying down for some time, just resting your mind and body. In this and all meditation exercises, note how you feel afterwards. Do you feel refreshed? Purified? Do you feel more or less negative emotion? Or do you feel much the same?

    Your feelings are clues to which practices are benefiting or harming you, or just wasting your time. But don't let that discourage you from sticking with a practice. Sometimes you have to carry on with it for some time before you begin to notice the effects.

15. After giving yourself some time, when your thoughts begin to return to your external world, open your eyes. Let yourself adjust for a bit. Then get up and resume your everyday activities with awareness.

Just as in a system of canal locks, the locks or gates are not all opened at once, so in this meditation, the chakras are only selectively opened. This allows the prana only to circulate between two or three chakras at a time. This creates closed, limited circuits. It side-steps the danger of of opening a complete circuit from root to crown, which could cause the kundalini to rise prematurely.

Remember that there are two phases in this meditation: first, bringing the energy up, step by step, from root to crown; and secondly, again pulling it back down to the root, step by step.

The second phase is essential. It grounds you by bringing the energy back into to the realm of everyday manifestation. You can't always hang out in the crown chakra or take a permanent vacation in the spiritual realm. You have to bring it back down to solid earth, to the world of everyday activity.

The second phase also allows you to clean out whatever residues the prana might have picked up when you were pushing and pulling it through the chakras. This cleanses the chakras and brings them into harmony with one another. It also facilitates healing. Even a small cut is subject to an infection, which needs to be emptied out and treated. Just so, when the chakras experience trauma, negative energy accumulates and festers. This meditation helps flush out the negative energy.

Healing the Chakras with Herbs

I'm sure you know that old proverb: An ounce of prevention is worth a pound of cure. But if you're already in need of a cure, sometimes the best remedy is not fast-acting, but slow and gentle. The meditations above might be too direct and aggressive an approach. Fortunately, there are gentler methods.

For millennia, the medical science of Ayurveda has been practiced in India as a way of healing the body and promoting a holistic, preventive approach to the health of body and mind. Ayurveda is concerned in part with the energy in the body and is a great supplement to practices that work with the chakras and the subtle energy system.

A number of herbs resonate with the energy of particular chakras and can be used to heal and balance them. I'll give a few choices for each chakra, because some of these herbs might be hard to find where you live. That goes especially for the Ayurvedic medicines, which may not be readily available in stores.

1. Herbs for the Root Chakra

Ayurveda: A great ayurvedic herb for remedying problems with the root chakra is **shilajit**. Shilajit is a pretty weird supplement, but it's very powerful and beneficial. It's a dark brown or black, tarry substance that oozes from between the rocks in the high Himalayas. It can also be found in the Caucasus and Altai mountain ranges.

As the Indian tectonic plate has pushed up against the Eurasian plate, it's caused the earth to buckle, raising up the great Himalayan mountain range. In the process, a lot of plant and vegetable matter was swallowed by the rocks. Over long centuries, it has transformed into the potent tarry substance shilajit.

Shilajit is full of minerals, vitamins, amino acids, and loads of natural compounds that are essential for good health. You can break off a small portion the size of a match head and mix it in with warm milk or water to drink.

If you can find shilajit, the purest quality freezes in cold weather and turns oozy when it's warm. You can test the quality by burning a small portion. If it expands and grows into ashy bubbles, it's pure.

General: Other herbs that help heal and balance the root chakra are cloves, dandelion, horseradish, and pepper. Root vegetables, such as potatoes and carrots, also support the root chakra. As these vegetables grow underground, they have a grounded, earthy energy that resonates with the root chakra.

2. Herbs for the Sacral Chakra

Ayurveda: A well-known aphrodisiac, **ashwagandha** (meaning, literally, "horse smell") has a reputation as "Indian viagra," but it has a lot more tricks up its sleeve than regulating sex drive. Ashwagandha is a root that is usually ground up and taken in capsule form. It increases your overall energy level—including, yes, your libido—but it also boosts the immune system and helps regulate mood. Specifically, it stabilizes serotonin levels, bringing them down if they're too high and raising them if they're too low. Since low serotonin is associated with anxiety and depression, ashwagandha is a great herb for treating these problems. It also regulates the stress hormone cortisol.

General: Calendula is an herb that helps to heal the sacral chakra and promote creativity. Other beneficial herbs are sandalwood, coriander, fennel, gardenia, cinnamon, and vanilla. Foods that promote healthy functioning of the chakra include meat, eggs, beans, and nuts.

3. Herbs for the Navel Chakra

Ayurveda: **Turmeric** is a common item in any Indian kitchen, but it's also an excellent home remedy and Ayurvedic medicine in its own right. The navel chakra, manipura, is connected to willpower, and also the digestive fire. Turmeric promotes healthy digestion by soothing or stimulating the digestive fire of the navel chakra as needed. It also helps reduce depression, which can dampen your willpower.

Turmeric often comes in powdered form. You can mix it with water and drink. A tablespoon of turmeric twice daily promotes good digestion. Some even swear it cures the symptoms of depression.

General: Mint, jasmine, lavender, rose, basil, andginger all help to heal the navel chakra. Pine pollen is also a potent healing agent for the navel chakra. It is full of DHEA, a substance which the body produces naturally. It enhances the adrenal glands and the endocrine system. It promotes self-confidence and willpower. It also improves digestion.

4. Herbs for the Heart Chakra

Ayurvedic: We already mentioned ashwagandha as an herb to heal the sacral chakra. Well, it's also very helpful for the heart chakra. Another herb that soothes and heals the heart chakra is **shatavari**. Shatavari is a general health tonic, which is also used specifically to support the female reproductive system. Here we're more concerned with how it encourages healthy functioning of the heart and supports the activity of the heart chakra.

It can be taken as a powder, in capsule form, or as a liquid. If you take it in powdered form, you can mix it with clarified butter. In that case, it's helpful to heat it in clarified butter to help release its healing properties.

General: Hawthorn berry, rose, and thyme all help to heal the heart chakra. Hawthorn berry especially has healing properties for the heart and helps treat heart problems such as arrhythmia and blood pressure. It's also a powerful antioxidant. It reduces stress and anxiety and promotes an emotional feeling of well-being and love.

5. Herbs for the Throat Chakra

Ayurveda: The throat chakra or *vishuddha* is connected with the thyroid gland. Any herbs that are used to treat thyroid disorders are also helpful for healing the throat chakra. The ayurvedic formula **kanchanara guggulu** is a potent remedy for problems with the thyroid gland. It removes stagnant phlegm from the body's tissues.

Also resonant with the throat chakra is **brahmi**. Brahmi is an herb that promotes concentration and cognitive functioning in general, and specifically speech and language. It's an excellent remedy for problems afflicting the throat chakra.

General: Peppermint, salt, and lemongrass are good herbs for treating throat chakra problems. Slippery elm can also be used to treat inflammations and irritations of the throat. Essential for thyroid health is a sufficient level of iodine in the body. Seaweed is full of iodine, as well as many other nutrients that are often lacking in modern diets.

6. Herbs for the Third Eye Chakra

Ayurveda: The third eye chakra is connected to the pineal gland and the higher functions of the brain. **Gotu kola** is a powerful ayurvedic herb for healing and enhancing this chakra. It increases oxygen uptake in the body's cells, and specifically and most importantly in the brain. It also thickens the corpus colossum, or tissue that connects the left and right hemispheres of the brain. This increases communication between the hemispheres and brings about an integration of intuitive and rational, holistic and linear styles of thinking. It also brings the right and left channels—ida and pingala—into harmony.

Meditators especially benefit from the use of this herb. It has been shown to increase intelligence in the long term.

General: In addition to eyebright, mugwort, poppy, rosemary, and lavender, passionflower is used to heal ailments of the third eye chakra. It treats insomnia, depression, anxiety, and headache, and improves mental clarity and cognition.

7. Herbs for the Crown Chakra

Ayurveda: The crown chakra is more rarefied and abstract than the other chakras. It is part of the subtle body system, but it's above and outside of the body. It acts as a gateway between the embodied and spiritual planes of our existence. So it needs an herb with a more subtle action.

Brahmi, mentioned earlier, in general promotes intelligence (and even hair growth) and works to heal the crown chakra. **Gotu kola** also works to heal this spiritual chakra. Both of these herbs aid focus and clarity, which allows you to ascend to higher levels in meditation.

There's also **shankh pushpi**. It reduces stress and keeps the mind in a relaxed, calm, focused state. It improves memory and promotes better sleep. In general, it induces a sense of peace and spiritual well-being.

General: Smudging herbs such as sage help cleanse the energy in the crown chakra, which facilitates better communication between the physical and spiritual parts of our being. Sage in particular has been shown to increase perceptual clarity, memory, healthy brain function, and intelligence.

Also helpful is lavender, which increases clarity, reduces anxiety, soothes the nervous system, and lowers depression. It also contains a number of antioxidant compounds.

A Parting Word

I have again and again stressed the dangers of jumping into practice without doing the proper groundwork, because I want to make sure the message gets hammered home. The dangers are real, and the spirituality scene is full of people who brought needless suffering upon themselves by their own carelessness. These warnings should not be taken as a discouragement from engaging in spiritual practice at all, but as an encouragement to enter into it cautiously and with the guidance of someone who knows what they're doing.

Since Eastern spirituality first burst in on the Western scene in a big way in the 60s, the word "guru" has become poisoned by its frequent abuse. A spiritual teacher does not have to be a cult leader or a shifty god-man. The Sanskrit word "guru" means "heavy," because an authentic guru is heavy with good qualities. So avoid the bad gurus like the plague and look for a guide whose genuine interest is in the spiritual growth of their students.

You now know enough about the chakras to get started. My hope for you is that you use the information in this book to explore your subtle body and mind in a safe way, find self-healing, and develop your spiritual practice into something deep and nourishing for your life.

Preview of Kundalini for Beginners

Introduction

→ Available on Amazon

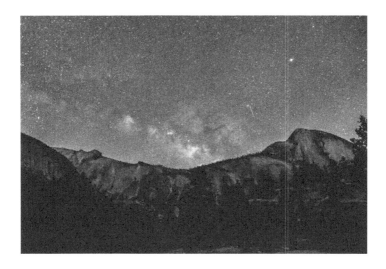

For several millennia, from a time stretching back into the dim reaches of prehistory, sages in India have dived deep into their own minds, attempting to uncover timeless spiritual truths. Through meditation, yoga, fasting, ascetic practice, renunciation, ritual, breath work, mantra, and creative visualization, these pioneers of the inner world have exerted themselves in the work of self-discovery, going deeper and deeper into their own experiences and psyches. Some of them have returned from this inner journey enriched and enlightened. These adepts managed to retrieve many treasures, which they passed on to students who, in turn, passed them on, until the present day. These treasures come in the forms of maps to our own minds, to the possibilities inherent in our experience. These maps outline the paths that we can take to achieve the same results as the masters of yore.

Of all these treasures, one of the most fascinating is the system of Kundalini yoga. At once mysterious and powerful, the idea of Kundalini—the so-called "serpent power" coiled at the base of the spine, waiting to be released—may seem like a distant, exotic fantasy. This book will aim to demystify this system of practice and make it intelligible.

What is Kundalini, and why awaken it? Put in simple terms, Kundalini is a dormant potential for spiritual transformation. When released, this potential explodes as a supernova of energy, which can have profound ramifications in all areas of one's life. She has the potential to lead to complete awakening and freedom from the conditioned, limited experience of ego— in other words, enlightenment. If you're reading this book, it's either because you have an inclination to the spiritual life or because you have experienced the arising of Kundalini yourself and are struggling to understand what it means and what to do about it. It is my hope that this book will have something to offer both kinds of readers.

To some extent, the contents of this book will overlap with those of *Chakras for Beginners*. This is unavoidable, as the system of esoteric anatomy outlined there is the background for the idea of Kundalini. When Kundalini is dormant, she is located in the root chakra of the subtle body and, when awakened, traverses the rest of the chakras in turn on her journey to the crown chakra.

It is important to have a grounding in the material of *Chakras for Beginners* before attempting to work on the material in this book. In general, the following progression of practice is recommended: yoga and meditation, followed by balancing the chakras, and only then arousing the Kundalini power.

Yoga and meditation are necessary to build a stable foundation for further practice. With yoga, you will train your body to be flexible and healthy, which prepares it for working with the subtle energy system through practices like pranayama. Your body will not be easily disturbed by sickness. Meditation will give you a steady and healthy mind with a powerful capacity for concentration, like an electron microscope pointed straight at your own being. Your mind will not easily be thrown off balance by emotional upheavals, nor will your psychological state be very affected by events and situations outside of your control.

Then, working with the chakras involves targeting specific areas of your psyche for balancing and healing. The chakra system is like a map of the psyche, which allows you to progressively clean up any impurities and heal old wounds. This is critical for working with Kundalini, because old *samskaras* or conditioning based on past traumas can throw you into the deep end when they meet with the rising force of Kundalini.

At all of these stages, it is beneficial to work under the guidance of a qualified teacher who can help you avoid pitfalls and dangers, as well as force you to work with the blind spots of your ego. But in the case of Kundalini especially, it is absolutely essential to have a teacher. So whatever is in this book should be viewed as a companion to a careful, responsible practice, rather than a substitute for a personal teacher.

There is no substitute for a living, breathing teacher. Maybe we think we can consult our inner teacher, or meet our teacher in dreams and visions. But we will only be fooling ourselves. To make any progress on the spiritual path and avoid the trap of getting caught in our own fantasy world, we cannot avoid the risk of being challenged by a teacher. It is only by means of such challenges that we can hope to win the result of the path.

What is Kundalini?

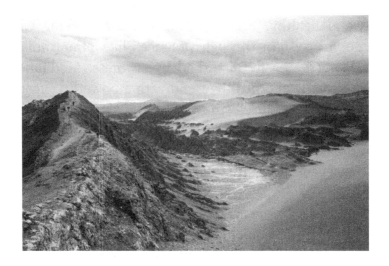

Kundalini is synonymous with Shakti, which literally means "power." In this case, we are talking about the innate divinity of the universe, which our sources call Shiva. His *shakti* is personified as a goddess. While Shiva is the supreme god, the source and transcendent witness of the phenomenal world, Shakti *is* that world itself. She is the ceaseless play of divine energy, the ongoing dance of phenomena. Together, Shiva and Shakti are the divine male and female modes of existence. But, in truth, they are not separate from each other, but an integral unity. This unity is also called *nonduality*.

This is not just metaphysical speculation or mythology. It's a description of your own experience, and is meant for you to understand at an experiential level. So the idea of Shiva and Shakti is not supposed to describe some remote state of affairs, but a very personal and intimate thing. It is an immanent reality, right now, the very dynamic of your own consciousness.

Subjectively, consciousness is experienced as two polarities. There is the consciousness itself, which has no particular color, shape, or attributes of its own, but simply reflects whatever it experiences. It is the eternal still point of awareness, changeless and untouched. At the same time, this consciousness manifests as the endless plurality, color, and fanfare of experience. This experience is both your own inner world and the world of your senses. That creative, energetic play of experience *is* Shakti, and your own still point of awareness *is* Shiva.

Nor are these poles separate things with an independent existence. The creative manifestation of experience is always happening within the changeless sphere of pure consciousness. That consciousness is the space within which our lives unfold.

Shiva is the ultimate Self and the ground of all being. Ultimately, we are identical with this Self. But he also takes individual, limited forms to explore the potential of his own being. The capital-S Self is not the same as the lowercase self of individual egohood. "Ego" is called *ahankara* in Sanskrit. It is that part of the self which thinks "me" and "mine," which tries to appropriate and possess experience, to freeze it into something solid and manageable, and which constructs elaborate stories and self-images. These thoughts are just that, thoughts—completely fictitious, with no more substance than a puff of smoke.

And yet they persist and have a powerful grip on us. Most of us live and die under ego's spell. We never get so much as a glimpse of what lies beyond the fictions that we spin about "I," "me," and "mine." The fabric of self-deception is woven from the filament of such thoughts. What possibilities would await us if we tore away that veil, if we unraveled this bewitchment?

Make no mistake, getting to that point is slow, painstaking work. It takes guts and a steely determination to work with your mind and experience, come what may. But somewhere along the way a breakthrough can occur. Your body and mind can suddenly be zapped by the energy of awakening, as if brought to life for the first time. It's not just an idea. It's a real possibility. That makes it both attractive and risky.

This can come about by conscious effort or by accident. In fact, the energy that we work with in Kundalini yoga is the very same energy that goes into the construction of ego. How could that be the case? When this energy is invested in protecting your personal identity and serving your own limited and selfish agenda, it manifests as ego. When it is awakened and aimed at spiritual liberation, it is known as Kundalini and quickly rises to meet its goal. So while awakening and egohood are opposite modes of being, the underlying reality that brings them to life is the same.

The spiritual path is not a matter of fixing yourself or "destroying" your ego as if you were something broken that needed to be replaced. The message of Kundalini is that your own present awareness, pristine and eternal, is already divine. Even egohood and negativity are just dynamic expressions of your inherent divinity. So the spiritual path is not about a process of making yourself better. It's about a process of preparing yourself for the recognition of the reality that already exists in the here and now.

This way of thinking unites the human and the divine, the transcendent and the immanent, permanent and impermanent, mind and body. It is quite alien to our usual Western way of understanding spirituality. In Western religions, individual humans are flawed, mortal creatures who are trying to relate to a perfect, immortal God who must remain forever separate from them.

Moreover, the legacy of modern thinking since Descartes has left us with a mind-body problem: how is this mind, which seems knowing and subjective, related to the physical body, which is objective, dumb, mechanical matter? This is not just a philosophical problem, but a cultural and personal one. It has to do with a modern malaise, our sense of alienation from ourselves. The responses to this have not been entirely satisfying: either deny the existence of the mental entirely and ascribe it to physical causes, or else hold on to mind-body dualism, the idea that somehow mind and body are separate things with independent existence.

The idea of Kundalini, with its nondual view, directly addresses this lacuna in the Western mindset. Your own consciousness is never separate from the richness of embodied experience. It is rather the source of all such experience. The various parts of your psyche map onto your subtle body, which acts as an intermediary between the gross physical body and the rarefied atmosphere of mind. The movement of subtle energies through the channels and chakras of the subtle body is the basis of the inner life of the mind. In the Kundalini worldview, which derives from Shaiva tantra, body and mind form an integral unity. Mind and body are just two ways of experiencing divinity. That's why many in the yoga community speak of a single *bodymind* instead of artificially separating these polarities of experience.

Kundalini and the Esoteric Anatomy

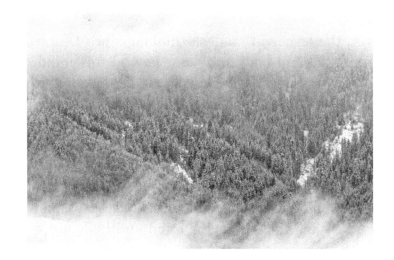

In order to arouse Kundalini, we must first understand how it fits into the esoteric anatomy, or subtle body system, of Indian yogic and tantric practice. While there are many such systems, the system we will work with is the most well-known one, the seven-chakra system.

In addition to the gross, material organs and constituents of the physical body, each of us also has a subtle body, which exists as an intermediary between the physical body and the psyche. This subtle body acts as both a support for different states of consciousness and as the interface by which the psyche interacts with the physical world.

The Channels

Woven throughout the subtle body like veins are thousands of *nadis* or channels. For our purposes, we will focus on three: *ida, pingala*, and *shushumna,* which run vertically through the body from the base of the spine to the crown of the head, intersecting at each of the first six chakras in turn.

- *Pingala* is the right channel, red in color. It's connected with the sun, the male principle, and has a heating effect. When it's active, our desires and passions increase, and we move towards sensory enjoyment.
- *Ida* is the left channel, white in color. It's connected with the moon, the female principle, and has a cooling effect. When it's active, it cools our passions, and we become relaxed and peaceful.
- *Shushumna* is the central channel, with neither color nor attributes. For most of us, who are under the spell of ego and external reality, this channel is not very active. It's like an empty road. But when Kundalini is awakened, *shushumna* is the route she will take to the *sahasrara* chakra at the crown of the head.

The Chakras

The points where these three channels meet are the six chakras. The seventh chakra, *sahasrara*, is not properly a chakra at all because it's not the intersection of more than one channel, being only the terminal point of the central channel. Still, it's included in the list of chakras as a seventh chakra because it's the final destination of awakened Kundalini. So it has pride of place.

The chakras are like a map to the human psyche, representing its development all the way from the lowest level of biological instinct to the highest spiritual achievement of enlightenment or awakening. In order from lowest to highest, representing the journey that Kundalini will take, the chakras are:

1. *Muladhara*, the root chakra located at the base of the spine or near the perineum. It's associated with the basic biological drive to survive. As such, it's connected with financial security, food, shelter, and feelings of safety. It's the instinct that makes you get food when you're hungry and money when you're broke.
2. *Svadhishthana*, the sacral chakra located just above *muladhara* near the sacrum bone. It's associated with sexuality and the reproductive instinct. It's also associated with the energy of libido in general. So it has to do not just with intimacy and erotic pleasure, but also any pleasure-seeking desire of a more basic kind.
3. *Manipura*, the navel chakra located just above the level of the navel. This chakra has to do with willpower, energy, and drive. At this level of development, we're talking about personal ambition and a well-developed sense of self-interest as opposed to mere instinct.
4. *Anahata*, the heart chakra located in the center of the chest (not exactly at the heart). This has to do with love, specifically meaning the ability to go beyond your own ego's interests in order to benefit other people. Everyone develops the first three chakras to some extent, even if dysfunctionally, but many people never really develop the heart chakra, only experiencing its energy on rare occasions or not at all.
5. *Vishuddha*, the throat chakra, is connected with speech, expression, art, creativity, and music. It has to do with a higher ability to communicate creatively.
6. *Ajña*, the "third eye" chakra, between the eyebrows and slightly above them, is connected with extremely penetrating intelligence, sudden intuition, mystical insight, and even psychic abilities. At this level you develop a very sharp, crystalline mental clarity.

7. *Sahasrara* or the crown chakra is located at the very crown of the head. This is identical to the highest Self, the individual's spirit or soul—pure, undifferentiated consciousness, eternal and untouched by the movements of the world. It has to do with nonduality and enlightenment. Spiritual enlightenment happens when the rising Kundalini reaches this chakra.

This is just the barest sketch of the subtle body system we're working with. All of these points are discussed in more detail in <u>Chakras for Beginners</u>, which gives a fuller understanding of the subtle body, how the chakras fit into it, and how you can start exploring them and working with their energy for healing and personal development.

Kundalini resides at base of the spine in the root chakra. She is said to be coiled there like a snake. She's coiled three and a half times around a lingam, which is a symbol of Shiva. The first three coils are the three *gunas*, which are like fundamental tendencies or phases of existence according to Indian philosophy. These gunas are called *sattva*, *rajas*, and *tamas*. *Sattva* has to do with harmony, equilibrium, and goodness, *rajas* with passion and activity, and *tamas* with chaos and stagnation. These are the modes that all manifest being takes.

The final half coil of Kundalini is the mouth of the serpent, ego. It's the serpent's mouth because of its poison. So while Kundalini is the means by which the aspirant transcends ego and ascends to the highest spiritual awakening, she is also the energy that undergirds ego—so long as she sleeps at the base of the spine. Kundalini is awakened when her energy, normally directed into maintaining the ego, is liberated and aimed instead at enlightenment. From *muladhara* she rises up to *sahasrara*, opening each of the chakras in turn, and finally unites with Shiva at the crown of the head. So ego's energy, once disentangled from its fictions, is freed to ascend to its loftiest goal, uniting in eternal bliss with the infinite source of all.

When Kundalini rises through the central channel, she opens each of the chakras in turn. Until she opens them, each of these chakras is closed, like a lotus that has not yet bloomed. As long as she resides in a chakra, it is open, like the petals of a fully blossomed lotus flower.

But before this happens, it's possible to do some preliminary work balancing and healing the chakras, as described in <u>Chakras for Beginners</u>. Still, it's the energy of Kundalini that fully activates the chakras and purifies them of any negative conditioning. If you haven't done the proper groundwork to prepare for this, to accommodate Kundalini's ascent through your system, her energy can be destructive and harmful. Later we will talk about some of the effects, both positive and negative, of Kundalini awakening.

The Five Pranas
There are 72,000 channels in the body, and subtle energy or *prana* moves through them. Prana enters and exits the body through nine doors: the two eyes, two ears, mouth, anus, and genitals. A yogi controls the movement of prana through the body, particularly in the *ida* and *pingala* channels. Through pranayama or breath control, he or she balances energetic activity of the left and right channels until they are equal. That way the energy can be induced to enter the *sushumna* and push Kundalini upward.

There are five kinds of prana in the body, which are also known as *vayu* ("wind"). These pranas regulate various physical functions and are important in the practice of Kundalini yoga.

1. *Prana-vayu* is the inward-moving energy that takes in everything from breath and food to sensory information and ideas. It governs the heart and lungs, and controls breathing and the beating of the heart. It comes into the body through the breath. It's located in the region of the heart and lungs. Here the "prana" of "prana-vayu" is a specific kind of energy and must be distinguished from prana or energy in the general sense.

2. *Apana-vayu* is the downward-moving energy that mainly functions to remove waste from the body as urine, feces, and menstrual blood. It also governs sex, because it moves energy down towards the genitals. So it also expels semen. Although it's located in the lower portion of the abdomen below the navel, it also expels air through exhalation.

3. *Udana-vayu* is the upward-moving energy, active mainly above the neck. It produces speech and governs consciousness and thought.

4. *Samana-vayu* is located between the heart and the navel. It's that energy which balances and processes. Here "processes" means things like digesting food and also absorbing oxygen in the lungs. It works in the mind to process our experiences.

5. *Vyana-vayu* is spread throughout the entire body. Its main jobs are to control all muscle movement and to circulate blood throughout the body.

For Kundalini yoga, the most important of these five pranas are the first two. The point here is that the prana-vayu and apana-vayu must be united through pranayama and yogic practice. Prana-vayu normally tends upwards, while apana-vayu normally tends to move downwards, in the direction of gravity. It also tends to pull consciousness down into worldly things, away from spiritual interests. So a practitioner has to reverse the usual flow of these two energies, making the apana-vayu move upwards and the prana-vayu downwards, so that they meet and unite. When that happens, they kindle a fire that stimulates Kundalini to awaken and rise up.

Preview of The Mindfulness Beginner's Bible

→ Available on Amazon

Chapter 1 - What is mindfulness?

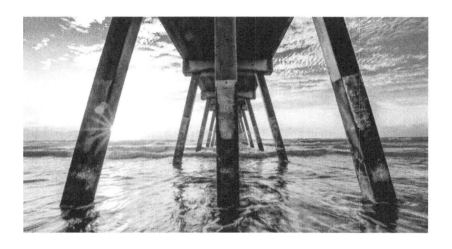

"Life is a dance. Mindfulness is witnessing that dance."
Amit Ray

Have you ever started eating a packet of chips and then suddenly realize that there is nothing left? This is one example of mindlessness that most of us experience on a daily basis. We, as humans often get so absorbed in our thoughts that we fail to experience what is happening right in front of us.

In modern society, most of us suffer from a condition called compulsive thinking. We have this hysterical inner voice that is constantly jumping from one thought to the next, obsessing about every little detail that could go wrong, complaining, comparing and criticizing everything and everyone. Sadly, most of us have become hostages to the whims of our minds, to the point where we even identify with the mind, thinking that we are our thoughts, when in reality we are the awareness behind our thoughts.

The moment you start observing your thoughts without identifying with them, you enter a higher level of consciousness beyond the mind and you reconnect with your true Self – the eternal part of you that is beyond the transient, ever-wavering physical realm.

Take a few seconds right now and become mindful of your hands. Feel the warmth that emanates from them. Rest your attention on every sensation in your hands. Feel your blood pulsing through them. Become one with your hands and notice the subtle tingling sensation as you become aware of them.

If you did this little exercise, I bet you noticed your mind becoming a bit more still. When you rest your attention on your body, you are living actively in the now. Awareness of the body instantly grounds you in the present moment and helps you awaken to a vast realm of consciousness beyond the mind, where all the things that truly matter - love, beauty, peace, creativity and joy - arise from.

Research has shown that we spend up to 50% of the time inside our heads - a state of mindlessness where we are continuously consumed by the chaotic impulses of our minds that are constantly thinking, ruminating the past and worrying about the future. Sadly, most people go through life in a walking haze, never really experiencing the present moment, which is our most precious asset.

Mindfulness is about being fully immersed into your inner and outer experience of the present moment. One of the best definitions of mindfulness is provided by the mindfulness teacher Jon Kabat-Zinn: "*Mindfulness means paying attention in a particular way; On purpose, in the present moment, and non-judgmentally.*"

Jon Kabat-Zinn breaks down mindfulness into its fundamental components: In mindfulness, our attention is held...

On purpose

Paying attention on purpose means intentionally directing your awareness. It goes beyond merely being aware of something. It means deliberately focusing your conscious awareness wherever you choose to, instead of being carried away in the perpetual storm of your thoughts.

Secondly, our attention is plunged...

In the Present Moment

The mind's natural tendency is to wander away from the present and get lost in the past or the future. Mindfulness requires being in complete non-resistance to the present moment.

Finally, our attention is held...

Non judgmentally

In mindfulness there is no judgment, there is no labeling, there is no resistance and there is no attachment. You simply observe your thoughts, feelings and sensations as they arise without ever energizing with them. As soon as you realize that you are not your thoughts, but the observer behind your thoughts, they will immediately lose power over your.

Mindfulness goes beyond basic awareness of your present experience. You could be aware that you are drinking tea, for example, however mindfully drinking tea looks very different. When you are mindfully drinking tea, you are purposefully aware of the entire process of drinking tea – you feel the warmth of the cup, the subtleties in smell and taste of the tea, the sensation of heat as you press your lips against the cup... – you intentionally immerse yourself in every single sensory detail that makes up the experience of drinking tea, to the point where you completely dissolve into the activity.

Mindfulness is about maintaining the intention of being completely plunged into your experience, whether it is drinking tea, breathing or doing the dishes. You can bring mindfulness to virtually any activity in your life.

Chapter 2 - The Power of the Present Moment

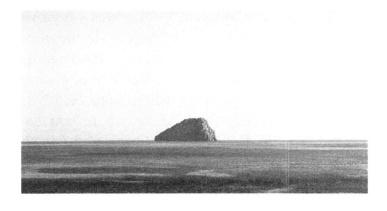

"I have realized that the past and future are real illusions, that they exist in the present, which is what there is and all there is."
Alan Watts

When you think about it, the present moment is the only moment that really exists. The past and the future are merely persistent illusions – the past is obviously over, and the future hasn't happened yet. As the saying goes, *"Tomorrow never comes"*. The future is merely a mental construct that is always around the corner.

Even when you dwell on the past or worry about the future, you're doing so in the present moment. At the end of the day, the present moment is all you and I have, and to spend most of our time outside the present means we are never truly living. Spiritual leader Eckhart Tolle puts it beautifully: *"People don't realize that now is all there ever is; there is no past or future except as memory or anticipation in your mind."*

However, most people spend most of their waking time imprisoned within the walls of their own thoughts, usually in regret of the past or in fear of the future, which are two ways of not living at all.

The present is the only moment in our lives where we have complete control over our destiny. We can decide our course of action only in the now – we can make a new friend, start a new business, get back to the gym, decide to stop smoking... The present is the only moment where your creative power can be exercised; it is the only place where you have full control over your life. Embracing the present moment is the only way to live a happier, healthier and more fulfilling life. As Buddha said, "*The secret of health for both mind and body is not to mourn for the past, worry about the future, or anticipate troubles, but to live in the present moment wisely and earnestly.*"

The biggest obstacle that keeps us from living in the present moment is the mind. Embracing mindfulness is a journey that requires practice and dedication, but it is a process that will inevitably lead you to a much happier and more fulfilling life where every moment is lived to the fullest. Here are 8 steps to start living in the present moment:

Practice non-resistance

The first step towards living in the present is learning to live in acceptance. You must learn to accept your life as it is today, rather than wish it was any other way. You must come into complete non-resistance with your current experience of life. By letting go of the hold the past has over you, you free your mind from unproductive thoughts and you reclaim the present moment. As Eckhart Tolle says, "*Accept - then act. Whatever the present moment contains, accept it as if you had chosen it. Always work with it, not against it.*"

Focus on the Now

In order to live in the present moment, you must focus on what you are doing in the now, whatever it may be. If you are doing the dishes, then do the dishes. If you're eating dinner, then eat dinner. Don't view the seemingly mundane activities in your life as nuisances that you hurry to get out of the way. These moments are what our lives are made up of, and not being present in them means we are not truly living.

Don't take your thoughts too seriously

Identification with the mind is the root of much unhappiness, disease and misery in the world. Most people have become so identified with their mental chatter that they become slaves to their own compulsive thoughts. Being unable to stop thinking and means we are never living in the present moment. When you learn to observe your thoughts as they come and go without identification, you step away from the chaotic impulses of the mind and you ground yourself in the now.

Meditate

You don't have to meditate to be mindful, but research has shown that engaging in a regular meditation practice has a spillover effect on the rest of your life. When you meditate you essentially carry the state of stillness and awareness that you experience during your meditation session into the rest of your day. Meditation is practice for the rest of your life.

Pay attention to the little things

Notice the seemingly insignificant things around you. Pay attention to nature for example. Notice the greenery around you - be grateful for every tree, every plant, every flower and realize that you could not survive without their presence. Go through your life as if everything is a miracle. From the majestic rising of the sun, to the chirping of birds outside your window, to the fact that your heart is beating every single second – life is truly a miracle to behold when you immerse yourself in the present moment.

Do one thing at a time

Multitasking is the opposite of living in the now. When your attention is divided between several tasks like eating, driving, making a phone call, you cannot fully experience the present moment. Studies have shown that people who multitask take about 50% longer to complete a task with a 50% larger error rate. To be more mindful, you must become a single-tasker. When you're eating, just eat. When you're talking to people, just talk to them. Develop the habit of being completely immersed into whatever you're doing. Not only will you be more efficient, but you'll also be more alive.

Don' try to quiet your mind

Living in the present moment does not require any special effort. The present moment is already at your fingertips. There is no need to expand energy to empty your mind. In mindfulness there is no stress, no struggle and no effort because you are not trying to force anything – you are in complete non-resistance to your current experience of life.

Stop worrying about the future

Worry takes you out of the present moment and in the future into an infinite world of possibilities. You cannot worry about the future and simultaneously live in the present moment. Instead of worrying about things that may or may not happen, spend you time preparing to the best of your ability and let go of the rest. Worrying won't change the future, but it will definitely elevate the cortisol levels in your body and drain you of your vital energy.

Made in the USA
Middletown, DE
10 September 2019